Your Personal Prescription Checklist

*How to Maximize Medication Safety
and Efficacy in the Age of Personalized Medicine*

Dr. Richard W. Snyder and Dr. Koroush Khalighi

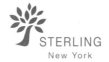

STERLING

New York

STERLING
New York

An Imprint of Sterling Publishing, Co., Inc.
1166 Avenue of the Americas
New York, NY 10016

ISBN 978-1-4549-1731-1

Distributed in Canada by Sterling Publishing Co., Inc.
c/o Canadian Manda Group, 664 Annette Street
Toronto, Ontario, Canada M6S 2C8
Distributed in the United Kingdom by GMC Distribution Services
Castle Place, 166 High Street, Lewes, East Sussex, England BN7 1XU
Distributed in Australia by Capricorn Link (Australia) Pty. Ltd.
P.O. Box 704, Windsor, NSW 2756, Australia

For information about custom editions, special sales, and premium and corporate purchases, please contact Sterling Special Sales at 800-805-5489 or specialsales@sterlingpublishing.com.

Manufactured in China

2 4 6 8 10 9 7 5 3 1

www.sterlingpublishing.com

DISCLAIMER
The information that is presented in this manual is for informational purposes and is not meant to replace or substitute for advice and treatment as determined by you and your doctor/health professional. We, the authors, are not directly involved in your medical care, and your medical situation may be different from those covered in this guide. We highly recommend discussion of this material with your doctor as it pertains to your own situation, and the information in this book should not be used as a substitute for your doctor's clinical judgment and opinion.

Contents

The Checklists

PROLOGUE

The Many Issues with Medications

As PHYSICIANS, ON A DAILY BASIS WE ARE WITNESS to the positive ways in which medications have not only improved our patients' life spans but also the quality of their lives. Pharmacologic interventions have been instrumental in the treatment of many widespread chronic conditions, including congestive heart failure, coronary artery disease, high blood pressure, and diabetes. However, it is important to remember that while medications can be lifesaving, they can also imperil our health when used improperly or in combination with one another or other substances.

According to a report from the American Medical Association, adverse drug reactions are a leading cause of death in this country, and approximately two million people per year experience some type of adverse drug reaction. According to a 2012 article from *Pharmacoepidemiology and Drug Safety*, about 20 percent of the population will likely have an adverse drug reaction, and an article from *Pharmacotherapy* reports that approximately 30 percent of all emergency room visits are medication related. This is nearly one out of every three emergency hospital visits. Even if you are already admitted to the hospital, you have a 17 percent chance of developing a serious drug reaction. Over 750,000 patients suffer from medication reactions on an annual basis once they are admitted to the hospital. In fact, adverse drug reactions remain a leading cause of increased morbidity and mortality in hospitalized patients.

The risk of developing a serious drug interaction increases exponentially depending on the number of medications you are taking. "Polypharmacy," which refers to the use of four or more different medications by one patient, is at epidemic proportions in the United States, especially among the elderly population. According to one study, the average adult over age sixty is currently taking an average of three or four medications that are being prescribed by more than one physician. Not only does the risk of adverse drug interactions rise with every added medication, but the risk of potentially fatal drug-drug interactions also dramatically increases.

Approximately half of all individuals in America are taking at least one or more medications that may not be needed. In 2013, over three billion prescriptions were filled for approximately three hundred million people, and most people likely took those medications without a second thought. In many ways, taking a prescription medication is like playing Russian roulette: For some people the side effects of these "beneficial medications" may be intolerable. For others, they may have no effect at all. For others still, prescription medications can directly cause harm or combine dangerously with other medications or supplements to cause harm. It is very difficult to predict how any given patient—with his or her unique metabolic profile—will react to any given medication.

I am a kidney doctor and have been practicing medicine for over a decade. My co-author, Dr. Khalighi, a cardiologist and electrophysiologist, has been practicing for even longer. On a daily basis, we see many people with complex medical problems, and the medication lists they bring to the office seem to get longer and longer with each and every visit. More medications means more potential for adverse drug reactions as well as drug-drug interactions. Then there are the plethora of herbal supplements and vitamins that patients take and may not tell their doctors about for fear of being criticized. In order to understand our purposes for writing this book, I would like to relate the following true story:

Mr. N is an older gentleman whom I have had the pleasure of knowing for years. He is married to a wonderful woman, Mrs. N, who is a staunch advocate for her husband's care. Her record-keeping and organizational skills are nothing short of phenomenal. She keeps a binder filled with information from doctor visits and pertinent lab data. She maintains an up-to-date medication list with notes and dates concerning dosage and medication changes, including which prescriber changed the medication and for what medical reason. In addition, she maintains a separate list with all of Mr. N's supplements and vitamins. Given his complex medical history, this is a necessity.

Mr. N has a significant history of heart-related illnesses. He has heart disease and has been hospitalized in the past for acute congestive heart failure. He has other chronic medical issues—including high blood pressure, diabetes, colitis, chronic congestive heart failure, chronic kidney disease, and gout—and has had a pacemaker and defibrillator implanted. His many medications include: losartan (Cozaar®), eplerenone (Inspra®), iso-sorbide mononitrate (Imdur®), aspirin, clopidogrel (Plavix®), and carvedilol (Coreg®) for his heart; insulin for his diabetes; febuxostat (Uloric®) for his gout; budesonide (Entocort®) for his colitis; and others. He is also taking a probiotic for his kidney disease and intestinal health and other supplements, including ubiquinone (coenzyme Q_{10}) and D-ribose for his heart and as natural energy boosters, in addition to omega-3 fish oil and vitamin D for inflammation reduction and bone health.

Mr. N easily takes at least ten to fifteen different pills and supplements on a daily basis, which is actually pared down compared to what he had previously been on. We had made a concerted effort to decrease the number of both supplements and medications he was taking. For example, we discontinued St. John's wort because it can harm the liver and make it break down some of his heart medications faster. During one visit, Mr. N was confused, which we felt may have been an effect of ropinirole, a drug for restless legs syndrome. Mrs. N was able to provide not only the date in which the medication had been prescribed but also the date in which Mr. N began taking it. The symptoms of confusion appeared soon after, so this medication was promptly discontinued, and a few days later he was back to his normal self.

While his quality of life is tremendous, credit needs to be given to his wife for her superhuman efforts, records, and organizational abilities concerning his medication and supplement regimen.

Heart disease, congestive heart failure, diabetes, stroke, emphysema, chronic obstructive pulmonary disease (COPD), and chronic kidney disease make up the majority of chronic medical conditions affecting millions of those in industrialized societies. Each of those chronic illnesses is associated with a plethora of prescribed medications, and each of those medications is associated with a host of side effects, drug interactions, and medication-induced nutritional deficiencies.

The medical establishment is making headway in increasing patient safety and enhancing patient understanding of their medications. The use of the electronic medical record (EMR) allows the prescriber to send accurate information on medications and dosages directly to the pharmacy, decreasing the risk of a mistake occurring because of a lost paper prescription or inscrutable handwriting. Most importantly, an EMR allows efficient and accurate communication between different physicians, nurses, and assistants involved in a patient's care. If a patient is coming to see me in the office for a checkup or consultation, I can see the results of other physician visits as well as an up-to-date medication list that includes new medications the patient may have been prescribed.

Hospitals are also improving their procedures with a special document called a "medication reconciliation form" that lists every prescription medication that must be "reconciled" with the medications administered or prescribed while you are in the hospital. Every time someone is transferred off the hospital floor for either a procedure or diagnostic test or transferred from one hospital floor to another, this form is printed and all medications are reviewed. When the patient is discharged from the hospital, the new medication list given to the patient is again "reconciled" with the medication list that they had from home when they first entered the hospital. (For more information concerning all aspects of hospital care, I urge you to read *The Patient's Checklist* by Elizabeth Bailey.) But even with all of the improvements described above, mistakes still happen. Keeping your own records and knowing the basics about how different classes of drugs interact with one another is so important.

The goal of this book is to help you "actively learn" about the medications that you are taking. Questions asked throughout this book will enable you to ask your health care provider more focused questions, and, through the use of checklists, this active learning exercise will become a personalized one as you check off the information that pertains to you. Approximately two-thirds of Americans take some form of an herbal supplement, and there are many herb-drug interactions that can have adverse outcomes. This book also seeks to provide some important information concerning supplements and herbs that people may consider using instead of or in conjunction with prescribed medications, so we have dedicated a chapter exclusively to this topic.

The field of "pharmacogenetics," which explores how inherited genetic differences in metabolic pathways affect a person's response to various drugs, is just beginning to take hold. Dr. Khalighi and I believe that this research should be able to provide prognostic information on not only the right medication but also the right dose for each individual.

What Does It Mean to Personalize Your Medication Prescription?

THE GOAL OF THIS SECTION IS TO HELP YOU fully understand what "personalized medicine" means and why it is vital to preventing adverse drug reactions. We believe that "personalizing" your medication regimen revolves around three key areas:

1 Understanding your own uniqueness with regard to how you may process medications

2 Understanding more about the medications you are taking, including side effects and potential drug interactions

3 Being aware of supplements used to treat many common health conditions and how to safely incorporate them into your personalized medication regimen

We have already mentioned that it can be difficult to predict how someone will respond to a medication. Let's say you have been diagnosed with essential tremors, a neurological disorder that causes you to shake uncontrollably. Your doctor writes a prescription for propranolol (Inderal®) at a low dose of 10 mg to be taken twice a day. Unlike other beta blockers, propranolol penetrates the blood-brain barrier and the same low dosage may have different effects in different people. For some, the frequency and intensity of the tremors will decrease, while others will require a higher dosage in order to achieve a therapeutic effect. Some people will have no reaction to this medication. Others may have mild depression and/or fatigue that worsens with higher dosages. Yet others will experience profound depression, fatigue, lethargy, and/or sexual dysfunction—all of which are common side effects with beta blockers at this dosage.

This variable response among individuals is attributable to differences in genetics and other factors, but our responses to medications can also evolve over time. Setting genetic differences aside, here are some key factors that can affect how our bodies react to a medication over a given period:

- *Body size and composition.* When you take a drug, it travels throughout the body and is diluted in the process. Smaller people may be more sensitive and require lower doses than larger people. In addition, some medications are lipophilic (fat soluble) and can be concentrated in body fat, reducing the concentration of the drug where you need it most. This means that a stable dosage may not have the same effects on patients if they dramatically gain or lose weight. Alternatively, many diseases such as hypertension and diabetes are worsened by obesity, and the need for medications to control them are reduced as weight loss occurs.

- *Conditions that affect our ability to absorb medications.* Most medications are absorbed through the stomach and small intestine, and several medical conditions impair the body's ability to absorb medications. Congestive heart failure (CHF), which you will read more about later on, occurs from the heart's inability to pump blood adequately or to relax adequately, and it can result in a build-up of fluid in the lungs, legs, and intestines. Diuretics can help control this fluid build-up, but they (and other drugs) are not absorbed well in patients with significant intestinal swelling, necessitating the use of intravenous diuretics until major swelling resolves. Diabetes is another condition that can affect the absorption of medications by damaging the nerve fibers that direct the movement of food throughout the stomach and intestines. This "diabetic gastroparesis" partially paralyzes the stomach and intestines, which wreaks havoc on the absorption of food and medication. Given the millions of people with CHF and diabetes, as well as the millions more with inflammatory bowel diseases such as Crohn's disease, individual variability in medication absorption is a very important factor for physicians to take into account.

- *Conditions that affect liver and kidney function.* Most medications are removed from the body by the liver or kidney. The liver can break down medications in the blood or eliminate them by pushing them into the intestines through the bile. The kidneys can filter out drugs from the blood and eliminate them via the urinary tract. Chronic alcoholism, hepatitis, fatty liver disease (which may impact up to 40 percent of patients), or damage from other medications like acetaminophen (Tylenol®) may affect the liver's ability to break down ingested substances normally. Further, conditions such as high blood pressure, diabetes, and congestive heart failure all can adversely affect kidney function as we get older. Worsening kidney function can decrease both the degree and the rate at which medications are eliminated from the body, which in turn increases the chance of developing adverse drug reactions and/or drug-drug interactions.

- **Being elderly.** The elderly have less muscle mass and may have more relative adipose tissue, absorption issues, and compromised liver or kidney function. Many health professionals use a creatinine blood test to help assess kidney function, but a lower body mass associated with aging can also produce a lower creatinine level. This can give the false impression to the clinician that the kidneys are functioning better than they really are, and necessary dosage reductions may not be made as a result, leading to adverse reactions. This is a significant problem, and special care must be taken when prescribing medications to elderly patients.

Pharmacokinetics and pharmacogenetics are the present and future of medicine. Pharmacokinetics determine how a given medication is absorbed, distributed, metabolized (processed or broken down), and eliminated by the body. The pharmacokinetics of every prescription drug is known, including how much is absorbed, how widely it is distributed in the body, where it is metabolized, and how it is eliminated. Unfortunately, pharmacokinetics are determined only in a small number of people who generally are healthy and of average body size. Pharmacogenetics is a field that explores how genetic differences help to determine how individuals may respond to a given medication. Genetic polymorphisms are small genetic variations that alter how well a drug will work in the body or how readily it can be metabolized or eliminated. Pharmacogenetic testing to examine these genetic polymorphisms is currently being performed for patients diagnosed with cancer or HIV to determine the best forms of therapy. However, millions of people are being prescribed medications for which their particular "pharmacokinetics" may be very different from those of "average" patients.

The main processing center for medications and many other substances in the liver is called the "cytochrome P450 (CYP450) system," which metabolizes drugs by placing an oxygen on them. Within this system are many different processing pathways called isoenzymes (e.g., CYP3A4, CYP2D6, CYP2C9, CYP2C19, and CYP1A2). The chemical structure of the medication determines whether it will penetrate an isoenzyme enough to be metabolized or not, and many drugs are metabolized by one—and *only* one—isoenzyme, so blocking that isoenzyme leads to higher blood concentrations of the drug. Blood tests can identify if a patient processes medications through an isoenzyme slower or faster than average. Understanding how a medication is processed by a particular pathway can help doctors avoid prescribing medications that would either inhibit the processing of other medications (increasing medication side-effect risk) or increase its metabolism (and decrease its effectiveness). *Believe it or not, medications can inhibit or increase the rate of metabolism of other medications by either speeding up or slowing down a particular pathway.* For example, certain antidepressants can slow the metabolism of medications that use the CYP2D6 pathway, such as certain commonly prescribed pain medications. And guess what? There have been reports of a very dangerous interaction between certain antidepressants and pain medications.

A Few Notes about the Testing

Much of this specialized testing may not be covered by your health insurance. However, there are labs that specialize in this type of testing, and due to the significant technologic advances, these tests are available to the consumer at a fraction of the cost of a few years ago. While personalized metabolic testing is not yet considered to be standard care, there are many health professionals who use these tests to help determine not only if the dosing of the medication is correct but also if the medication itself needs to be changed. With major technological advances in basic sciences, genetic information will be increasingly available to everyone. More likely than not, physicians will embrace genetic-information-based personal medicine as a routine for daily practice in the near future.

....

THE PERSONALIZED APPROACH
A Study

Dr. Koroush Khalighi is a cardiology and clinical researcher who has extensively studied metabolic testing. Warfarin (Coumadin®) is one of the most commonly prescribed blood thinners for the treatment of medical conditions including atrial fibrillation (an abnormal rhythm of the heart) and deep venous thrombosis. It is also one of the most common medications for which a person can develop a potentially fatal adverse drug reaction: internal bleeding.

Dr. Khalighi and his team presented research at the World Congress of Cardiology in 2014 about the personalized pharmacokinetic testing results of over 300 individuals taking warfarin. Out of 301 patients tested, 190 patients were found to metabolize these medications normally, 104 demonstrated intermediate metabolism, and 10 were slow metabolizers. These same patients were also tested in order to determine their sensitivity (i.e., risk of bleeding) to the drug. Based on genetic testing, 109 patients were found to have low sensitivity, 145 had intermediate sensitivity, and 50 patients were extremely sensitive. Patients who were found to be intermediate metabolizers needed a 33 percent dose reduction, and those with low sensitivity needed their dosage increased by 33 percent, compared to those who metabolized through this pathway "normally."

Warfarin dosage adjustments, which were based on the results of pharmacokinetic testing, prevented significant adverse reactions from occurring. In addition, the use of genetic testing also helped to identify those patients who were at increased risk of developing toxicity and who required closer monitoring.

This study shows that if you are especially sensitive to the effects of warfarin as well as being a slow metabolizer (you process this medication slowly), you will need to start at a very low dose of this medication, while a fast metabolizer with low sensitivity to this medication may need a higher dose to begin with. Thus, pharmacokinetic testing can help to lower bleeding events without compromising clinical efficacy.

....

There is much more to learn and understand about personalized medicine, but it can confer a huge health advantage to ask yourself and your doctor, "Should I have pharmacogenetic testing before taking these medications?" We believe the answer is yes, especially if you are taking a few medications with a higher propensity for adverse drug reactions and interactions, such as blood thinners.

It is important to remember that, while the use of this type of testing can provide a "blueprint" for how you may process medications, the results can differ among individuals. That being said, the testing offers physicians some direction as to which medications may be better and safer compared with other types. In this book, in addition to providing you with a framework for understanding the basics of the most commonly prescribed medications, we also will include any known information pertaining to genetic testing and how these medications are processed in the liver.

Personalizing the Medical Regimen with Supplements and Natural Agents

Personalizing a medication regimen means more than pharmacokinetic testing; it involves understanding all of the therapeutic options available to you. While I am a kidney doctor, I have incorporated a few natural agents into my clinical practice for several years and feel comfortable discussing and integrating certain supplements into a comprehensive, personalized medication plan. I would like to let health professionals in on a little secret: patients and their families want to discuss these options with you without having their questions or concerns dismissed. This is why we have included in this book specific supplements that can be considered for certain medical problems.

If you go back to the example at the beginning of this book, Mr. N takes medications and supplements, and he can personally vouch for the efficacy of the supplements he is taking. With the use of D-ribose, he attests that his energy level has increased tremendously. He has been able to participate in an exercise program involving not only free weights but also aerobic training, which has further helped his heart condition. His overall state and demeanor have improved along with his energy level, and for this reason, Mr. N represents a personalized-medicine success story.

How to Use This Book

THIS BOOK, WHILE NOT AN EXHAUSTIVE RESOURCE ON ALL medications, provides an overview and interactive guide that will help you gain a perspective on the medications you are taking and empower you to be your own health advocate. Medications are listed with their generic name, often followed by the most common brand name of that generic.

The first checklist will give you basic questions to ask your doctor when you are being prescribed a medication, and the rest of the checklist chapters will deal with "medication classes"—groups of medications often prescribed to treat a particular medical condition or a disease process. While there are countless classes of medications, we chose to focus on the medications most commonly prescribed by physicians and other health professionals. The use of checklists in different aspects of medicine has been critical to organizing information, improving care, and making sure no stone is left unturned. Hospitals use checklists for the treatment of many conditions, including pneumonia, congestive heart failure, and chest pain. It improves the efficiency of care, with a focus on patient safety.

Checklists can also be effective learning tools. For the rest of this book, you will be reviewing the medication checklists (and checking off the relevant information) to help you better understand the medications you have been prescribed, or those that your doctor may have spoken with you about. The use of these checklists also serves to:

- Help you ask pertinent questions concerning your medications, including possible side effects and reasons for prescribing

- Enable you to understand possible nutrient deficiencies incurred by a medication or class of medications

- Keep track of your prescription and symptom history, helping you to draw connections between them

- Create your own "medication and supplement diary" that you can update and take with you to each of your doctor appointments

Discussion of "pharmacokinetic profiling" will be included where applicable. There are some classes of medications for which personalized testing is utilized to achieve optimal dosage, while other classes have not yet been studied extensively enough to provide information that would be useful for profiling.

Checklist Summaries

Checklist 1: The Essential Questions

This introductory chapter presents the most important considerations that doctors and patients need to take into account before prescribing or taking medications and/or supplements of all kinds. From possible nonpharmacologic options to knowing when to call your doctor, this checklist helps you to develop a "big picture" perspective on your medical treatment.

Checklist 2: Cholesterol Medications

In addition to reviewing the different classes of cholesterol- and lipid-lowering medications, this chapter will examine the debate concerning statin therapy and personalized testing concerning your cholesterol profile. Does a high cholesterol number necessarily warrant initiating statin therapy? In addition, we explore what other types of medications might be appropriate options based on your particular pharmacokinetic profile.

Checklist 3: Heart & Blood Pressure Medications

The leading reasons that people are admitted to the hospital are heart-related problems, including heart disease and congestive heart failure. Many heart and blood pressure medications including beta blockers, nitrates, calcium channel blockers, and others will be discussed in this chapter.

Checklist 4: Warfarin & Other Blood Thinners

Blood thinners increase the risk of developing side effects, including life-threatening bleeding in the GI tract, urinary system, and brain. We have seen patients admitted to the hospital for dangerous bleeding episodes too many times. The use of warfarin and other blood thinners also has the propensity to interact with many other medications. Clopidogrel (Plavix) and many of the newer antiplatelet medications will also be discussed.

Checklist 5: Medications & the Psyche

This chapter covers medications prescribed for the treatment of seizures, depression, psychosis, and anxiety. Antidepressants, including widely prescribed SSRIs, as well as benzodiazepines and antipsychotics will be discussed.

Checklist 6: Diabetes Medications

Diabetes is a growing epidemic responsible for eye, heart, kidney, and nerve problems, and there is a whole host of medication classes prescribed to combat its symptoms and effects. We review the pharmacokinetics of these medications in this chapter.

Checklist 7: Heartburn & GI-Related Issues

Gastrointestinal issues, including heartburn and belly pain, are some of the most common reasons that patients see their doctor. This chapter reviews the pros and cons concerning the use of medications such as histamine (H_2) blockers and proton-pump inhibitors, especially on a long-term basis.

Checklist 8: Treating Pain

Millions of Americans suffer from pain from multiple causes, including arthritis and chronic illness. Both prescription and nonprescription painkillers are not without side effects. This chapter reviews the common medications prescribed for chronic and acute pain, including opiates and nonsteroidal anti-inflammatory medications.

Checklist 9: Antibiotics

Millions of antibiotics are prescribed every year. There are many different classes, but our goal is to focus on only the most common ones.

Checklist 10: Natural Supplements

In this chapter, we review many commonly used supplements as well as the data concerning how they are processed by the liver. One of the best examples of this concerns vitamin D: those who are fast metabolizers of certain liver-processing pathways and those who are taking certain medications are prone to lower levels of this vitamin.

* * *

Following the checklists, several sections allow you to track important information as you navigate the healthcare system, including:

- Doctor Visits & Test Results

- Medication List

- Supplement List

- Doctor Contacts

Finally, toward the end of this book, a **Resources** section lists useful websites and organizations that can help you learn everything there is to know about various classes of medications and receive personalized testing. This is followed by a **References** section that provides sources for the information in each chapter, including peer-reviewed medical journals in case you would like to learn more about certain medications, studies, and other findings related to pharmacokinetics.

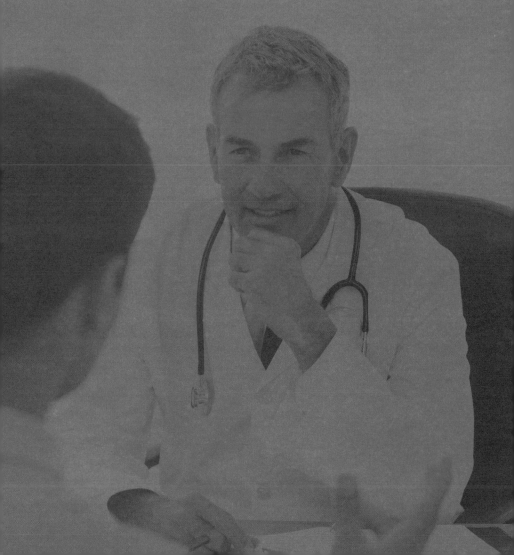

The Essential Questions

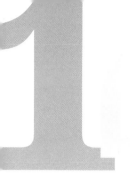

The Essential Questions

THIS CHECKLIST HAS SEVERAL BASIC QUESTIONS THAT ARE IMPORTANT to ask your doctor when you are being prescribed any medication. These questions will help you and your physician make the best decisions for your health, including proper precautions based on your medical history. They will also help you understand which side effects are common and less serious, and which require immediate medical attention.

1. ☐ Why has this particular medication been prescribed?

_____

_____

- Medicine is both an art and a science, so it is important to understand your physician's thought process, including why he or she thinks a particular medication's therapeutic benefit outweighs the potential for side effects in your individual case.

- Understanding why you are taking a medication increases the likelihood that you will start taking the medication and stick with it.

2. ☐ Are there any nonpharmacologic options for combatting this condition that I can undertake in lieu of or in addition to this medication?

_____

_____

- While medication can be effective in the treatment of an acute or chronic medical condition, being aware of your nonpharmacologic options can be just as important. While such options may not completely eliminate the need for medication, they may reduce the dose of the medication, which in turn can decrease the risk of adverse drug reactions, drug-drug interactions, and side effects.

- For example, medications commonly prescribed for the treatment of chronic pain can be very effective, but they also have significant side-effect profiles. Understanding nonpharmacologic options—including dietary changes, exercise, yoga, massage, and supplements that can reduce inflammation—may not only decrease the dose of the medication but also potentially eliminate the need for chronic pain medication altogether.

3 ☐ **What if I have not done well when prescribed other similar medications in the past?**

- If you have suffered from side effects or an adverse reaction to a medication in the same class as the one being prescribed now, discuss this with your doctor, who can then look into prescribing another class of medication. For example, statins are a medication class used to treat high cholesterol. Sometimes, after someone is prescribed a statin, he or she may encounter severe muscle and joint aches that may require discontinuation of the medication. If another doctor previously prescribed a statin medication that you could not tolerate, your current doctor should consider another class of cholesterol-lowering medication.

- This question also offers you a chance to discuss medication allergies. For example, if a person has an allergic reaction to a penicillin, he or she may be prescribed one of the "cephalosporins," but it is important to note that there can be some cross-reactivity between these medications—i.e., a small group of individuals with hypersensitivity to penicillins have an increased risk of developing an allergic reaction to cephalosporins—so most physicians will prescribe another class of antibiotics if possible, given the prior history. (Note: If the nature of the "reaction" you had was "stomach upset," then this is not a true allergy.)

- The take-home message is this: Know what medications you have not tolerated well in the past, and ask your doctor if there may be some overlap between those and the medication you are being prescribed now.

Allergic Reactions vs. Adverse Reactions

When asked by their doctor, "Are you allergic to any medications?" many people confuse adverse reactions with allergic reactions. For example, someone with a true allergy to penicillin may have symptoms that include hives (an early sign of allergy) or anaphylaxis (swollen tongue or swelling of the face). Anaphylactic shock is a serious medical condition that can cause loss of blood pressure and has a high morbidity and mortality rate if not recognized early and promptly treated. By contrast, an adverse drug reaction to penicillin can include stomach upset, diarrhea, and/or flu-like symptoms. This is why your doctor will ask you not only if you are allergic to any medication but also the nature of the allergy. If you say that when you took penicillin, you broke out in hives, chances are that your doctor will not prescribe it. However, if you had only mild stomach upset, this is an adverse reaction that is not life threatening. If your clinical condition warrants this medication, your doctor may prescribe it anyway, along with tips on how to minimize the risk of stomach upset (e.g., taking the medication after a meal), since not taking the medication could result in a much worse outcome.

* * *

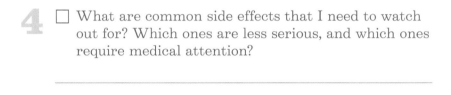

4 ☐ What are common side effects that I need to watch out for? Which ones are less serious, and which ones require medical attention?

_____

_____

- While there are any number of side effects (aside from allergy symptoms) that one can experience while taking a medication, we physicians are very cognizant of the most common possible side effects that people may experience. For example, the most common side effect of ACE (angiotensin-converting enzyme) inhibitors, which are prescribed for the treatment of high blood pressure and congestive heart failure, is a cough. If you experience this side effect, your doctor may discontinue this medication—especially if the cough is severe and persistent—but if your cough is only mild and intermittent, watching and waiting might be a better alternative, as this medication class has significant heart-protective effects. The important thing is keeping an ongoing dialogue with your doctor.

5 ☐ Does this medication require any type of blood testing once I begin taking it to ensure the dose is safe and therapeutic? What are the symptoms and consequences of overdose?

- Some medications require monitoring their levels in the blood to ensure the medication dosage is at the right therapeutic level. Being over this "therapeutic blood level" increases the risk of developing toxic side effects.

- Common examples of medications that require such blood-level monitoring include the heart drug digoxin (Lanoxin®), the asthma drug theophylline (Theo-Dur®), the mood stabilizer lithium (Eskalith®), and the anticonvulsant phenytoin (Dilantin®).

- Other medications require different types of blood monitoring related to the action of that medication. For example, diuretics and ACE (angiotensin-converting enzyme) inhibitors are prescribed for the treatment of high blood pressure, and routine monitoring of your kidney function is important when taking them because, while they have positive effects on blood pressure, they increase the risk of developing acute kidney faliure and may also raise potassium levels to dangerous levels, affecting the heart.

- It is also important to be aware of the signs and symptoms of overdose for any medication you take. It is possible to take too much of any medication, though some are easier to overdose on than others, and some overdoses are more serious than others. Being aware of signs and symptoms of overdose is especially important when taking medications that affect brain chemistry. For example, a lithium overdose is a medical emergency for which hospitalization is needed, and in severe cases dialysis is required in order to remove the lithium from the body and prevent permanent neurologic sequelae.

Understanding the Basic Blood Tests

In the following chapters, reference is made to particular blood tests that health professionals need to order if you are on certain medications, such as statins. For example, blood testing can indicate if you have anemia or any kidney or liver issues. *It goes without saying that you should always keep a copy of your blood work, and don't hesitate to ask your doctor to provide one.*

- *Complete Blood Count (CBC):* This test measures your white cell count (which, when elevated, may indicate infection or inflammation); your red blood cell count, hemoglobin count, and hematocrit (the volume of red blood cells in the blood, which, when lowered, may indicate anemia); and platelet count (which indicates how easily your blood clots).
- *INR:* This stands for "international normalized ratio," and the test is used to measure how thin or thick your blood is (e.g., how long it takes to clot) if you are taking the blood thinner warfarin. Clotting time might also be prolonged if you have advanced liver disease, meaning that the liver's blood-clotting ability is compromised. A related test, usually done in a hospital setting, is partial thromboplastin time (PTT), which tells health professionals how thin your blood is after a continuous, intravenous infusion of heparin.
- *Creatinine:* Your kidneys function as the body's filters, and measuring serum creatinine is an indirect way for your doctor to determine the "glomerular filtration rate" (GFR), which indicates how well your kidneys are working. Basically, the lower your serum creatinine, the better your kidneys are at clearing it from the bloodstream. It is important to have a sense of your kidney function prior to starting any medication, as it can impact not only the type of medication prescribed but also the dosage of many medications. For example, the medication spironolactone (Aldactone®) is commonly prescribed for the treatment of heart failure, but if a patient's GFR is less than 25–30 percent, alternatives should be considered. Certain antibiotics, such as Bactrim, cannot be prescribed if the kidney function is less than 30 percent in order to prevent further damage to the kidneys.
- *Liver Function Tests:* The proper functioning of the liver is important for the majority of medications—especially statins. Specific liver tests your doctor might order include assessments of aspartate aminotransferase (AST) levels and alanine aminotransferase (ALT) levels. If these levels are elevated, your doctor may need to adjust your medication dose and/or discontinue it. Other tests that are part of a " liver function panel" include bilirubin level and alkaline phosphatase level. If these levels are elevated, that may indicate

liver dysfunction, although problems with the gall bladder and biliary system can affect these levels as well.

* * *

6 ☐ Will this medication interact with any medications that I am currently taking? Which supplements, food, and beverages should I avoid?

_____

_____

- This is an important question to ask your doctor. If your physician is not entirely certain of all the potential interactions between different medications, supplements, and foods, then ask your pharmacist, who has access to information that can help determine if you are at risk of significant adverse interactions. If you look in the Resources section of this book, you will see links to useful websites where you can do your own research.

- Common dietary supplements can interact with many classes of medications. Examples include grapefruit juice and St John's wort, which can affect the processing of many medications in the body and increase the risk of adverse drug reactions.

- As the processing of many of the medications in this book is affected by liver function, it is a very good idea to minimize the use of alcohol if you are taking prescription medications. The combination can be dangerous or even lethal depending on the nature of medication(s) prescribed.

* * *

DOCTOR'S SPOTLIGHT

Grapefruit—Medication Interactions

Whether you are taking an over-the-counter medication or a prescription medication, it is very important to consider how they might interact with other substances that might be a part of your diet or lifestyle. One seemingly benign part of a healthy diet—grapefruit—actually contains chemical compounds called furanocoumarins that can have very serious effects on the metabolism of many common drugs (especially those metabolized by CYP3A4). Below is an incomplete list. _Before taking any medication, be sure to verify with your doctor whether or not it is safe to consume grapefruit or grapefruit juice._

- *Erythromycin:* Drinking grapefruit juice while taking this antibiotic can result in rapid heartbeats, which can potentially lead to sudden death.
- *Statins:* The combination of grapefruit with cholesterol-lowering statins— particularly simvastatin (Zocor®) and lovastatin (Mevacor®)—could potentially result in rhabdomyolysis (rapid muscle breakdown), which in turn can cause serious kidney damage.
- *Certain heart medications:* Grapefruit combined with antiarrythmics such as amiodarone (Cordarone®) can also cause rapid heartbeat and possible sudden death, and combination of grapefruit with calcium channel blockers (CCBs) such as verapamil (Calan®) can lead to fatal heart block. Further, if you are taking diuretics like eplerenone (Inspra) for heart failure or high blood pressure, you also need to avoid grapefruit, which increases the risk of high blood potassium levels and heart arrhythmias.
- *Certain blood thinners:* Combining apixaban (Eliquis®) or antiplatelet agents like ticagrelor (Brilinta®) with grapefruit can increase gastrointestinal bleeding risk.
- *Dextromethorphan:* Found in many over-the-counter cough and cold medicines, this drug can depress respiration (i.e., breathing) when combined with grapefruit.
- *Opioid painkillers:* Taking potent narcotics like fentanyl (Duragesic®) or oxycodone (OxyContin®) with grapefruit can result in potentially fatal respiratory depression.
- *Cyclosporine:* This medication can suppress the immune system and is prescribed to patients with solid organ transplants. Combining cyclosporine with grapefruit can increase blood levels of the medication, which increases the risk of a severely depressed immune system and worsened kidney function.

* * *

☐ Are there any nutritional deficiencies induced by this medication?

_____

_____

- Many medications have the potential to cause nutritional deficiencies that may require monitoring and replacement. Common examples include: B_{12} deficiency caused by metformin (Glucophage®), a commonly prescribed medication for type 2 diabetes; low potassium and magnesium levels caused by diuretics; and really low magnesium levels and vitamin D malabsorption caused by proton pump inhibitors (PPIs), used for the treatment of heartburn and ulcers.

8 ☐ What happens if I decide not to take this medication?

_____

_____

- As with any prescribed treatment, you have the right to decide to take or not take the medication suggested by your doctor. The best that we physicians can do is provide the information you need to make the decision for yourself or for your family member.

9 ☐ What if I am pregnant or become pregnant during the course of treatment?

_____

_____

- *If you are pregnant or are planning to get pregnant, make this clear to your physician.* All of your prescribed medications need to be evaluated with this in mind. Many medications (usually referred to as a "Category C, D, or X" in many drug reference books and websites) have the potential to cause birth defects. For example, if you are thinking of becoming pregnant, you must stop any statin (listed under "Category X") a few months before trying to conceive.

10 ☐ What should I do if I miss a dose?

_____

_____

- If you a miss a dose and have not received prior instruction about what to do, call your doctor or pharmacist. What you don't want to do in this situation is automatically double up on the medication when you take the next dose, as this can cause an adverse effect in some instances. For example, let's say that your day is hectic and you miss the morning dose of your blood pressure medication. If you take a double dose in the afternoon, it may drop your blood pressure too low.

- In general, if you miss a dose of a medication, nine times out of ten, you are going to be OK. However, with blood thinners (especially warfarin), it pays to be smart about it and give your doctor a call.

Notes

Cholesterol Medications

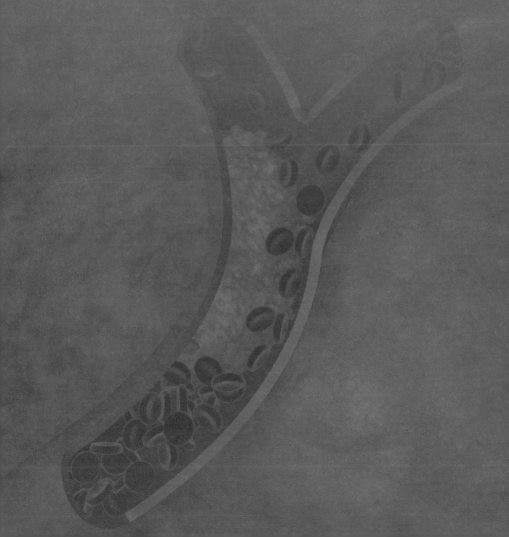

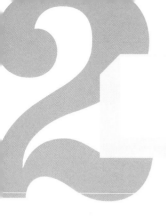

Cholesterol Medications

MEDICATIONS TO TREAT HIGH CHOLESTEROL AND TRIGLYCERIDE LEVELS ARE among the most commonly prescribed drugs. The medications discussed in this chapter are effective for lowering these levels, but as with other medications in this book, there are side effects and drug interactions of which you need to be aware.

Cholesterol is an essential lipid molecule synthesized in our bodies for the purpose of maintaining the structural integrity and fluidity of cell membranes. There are different "components" of cholesterol, including low-density lipoprotein (LDL), which is associated with the accumulation of plaques within arteries that can restrict or block blood flow, leading to heart attacks and stroke. Many, if not all, of the medications in this chapter work by different mechanisms to lower these "bad cholesterol" levels. High-density lipoprotein (HDL), on the other hand, is often referred to as the "good cholesterol," and higher HDL levels are considered heart protective, since those lipoproteins are believed to reduce arterial blockages. A total blood-cholesterol concentration above 200 milligrams per deciliter (mg/dL) is associated with an increased risk for developing heart disease, which is the leading cause of morbidity and mortality in industrialized nations, although higher HDL concentrations relative to LDL concentrations are believed to reduce this risk.

Statins are one of the most popular classes of medications. They work by blocking steps that are important for the production of cholesterol. While statin medications are very similar as a class, there are some differences among the specific medications. Commonly prescribed statin medications include atorvastatin (Lipitor®), simvastatin (Zocor), rosuvastatin (Crestor®), and pravastatin (Pravachol®).

When a statin medication fails to lower cholesterol levels enough and/or a patient is found to be intolerant of the drug, physicians may explore other options. These options include **ezetimibe (Zetia®)** and a class of medications called **bile acid sequestrants**—both of which work by blocking the absorption of cholesterol in the intestine.

Last but not least, in the summer of 2015 the medical community was introduced to a new class of cholesterol-lowering medications: the **PCSK9 inhibitors**. These represent yet another weapon in the armamentarium that physicians have for lowering cholesterol levels to what your range should be depending on your own particular own health situation. If you have documented heart disease or have risk factors for heart disease, many clinicians aim to reduce your LDL levels to 100 or below. Newer studies combining statins with either ezetimibe (Zetia) or PCSK9 inhibitors have aimed for LDL levels below 70 mg/dL.

A triglyceride is another type of lipid that circulates in the bloodstream, supplying cells with energy. Some of these triglycerides are packed into very low–density lipoproteins (VLDLs), and higher concentrations of this, along with LDL, can accelerate heart disease. However, very high triglycerides can also induce pancreatitis, a very serious inflammation of the pancreas. **Fibrate** medications such as gemfibrozil (Lopid®) and fenofibrate (TriCor®) are first-line agents prescribed to help lower triglyceride levels and can be combined with statins, niacin, or omega-3 fish oil for additional lowering.

Before we proceed, we need to reiterate a point that you will see again in upcoming chapters: *diet and exercise should be the first form of therapy for the treatment of high cholesterol levels.* If you are unable to decrease your cholesterol and/or triglyceride levels to healthy levels despite reforms to your diet and exercise regimen, or if you have other risk factors for heart disease, then your doctor may prescribe one or more medications.

THE PERSONALIZED APPROACH

Cholesterol Testing

In addition to risk factors and cardiac-risk-scoring calculators discussed later in this chapter, the use of personalized cholesterol testing—called the vertical auto profile (VAP) test—may also be an effective tool for determining the type of cholesterol medication you should be prescribed. Although not yet considered a standard of care, this type of testing goes above and beyond traditional cholesterol testing in determining a patient's cholesterol profile.

Traditional blood testing involves measuring the total levels of cholesterol, LDL, HDL, and triglycerides. VAP testing is a specialized blood test that takes cholesterol testing to a whole new level. It can help you to determine subtypes of your HDL and LDL particles and can even help determine your "atherogenic risk" (risk of developing heart disease) based on those particles. For example, short, dense LDL particles are thought to represent a larger atherogenic risk compared to the fluffy type of particles. The goal of this type of testing is not to focus on cholesterol as a number to be lowered, but rather to personalize treatment.

Let's say that on routine blood testing you were found to have a LDL level of 160 mg/dL. This level would prompt many physicians and health professionals to initiate treatment with a statin. If further VAP testing demonstrated that your cholesterol was fluffy and less dense, however, this would mean that the atherogenic potential of this cholesterol would be less than if the lipid particles were smaller and denser. Thus, VAP testing may help determine whether or not a person with borderline or high levels of cholesterol actually requires statin therapy.

....

Statins

Of all the classes of medications, the statins are among the most studied. In addition to treating high cholesterol levels, research studies have demonstrated that they have heart-protective effects, and they are considered the standard of care if someone has heart disease or significant risk factors for developing this condition. These factors include high cholesterol levels, diabetes, high blood pressure, and a strong family history of heart disease.

The following questions are intended to help you and your doctor determine which cholesterol medication(s), if any, is best for you and decide if anything about your regimen needs to be adjusted now or down the line. These questions will also help you better understand your medication(s) as well as track side effects and reactions.

1 Which (if any) of the following statins are you currently taking?

☐ Rosuvastatin (Crestor)

☐ Atorvastatin (Lipitor)

☐ Fluvastatin (Lescol®)

☐ Simvastatin (Zocor)

☐ Pravastatin (Pravachol)

☐ Pitavastatin (Livalo®)

☐ Other: _____

2 What dose are you currently taking, at what frequency?

_____ mg _____ times a day.

- Some cholesterol medications—including pravastatin (Pravachol), lovastatin (Mevacor), and fluvastatin (Lescol)—should be taken at night to maximize their impact on blocking cholesterol production. Other statins can be taken any time of the day, since they have a longer half-life (i.e., they stay in the body longer).

- Simvastatin dosing starts at 10 mg and intervals can increase to 20 and 40 mg daily; atorvastatin starts at 10 mg and can be dosed 20, 40, and

80 mg daily; pravastatin also starts at 10, 20, and 40 mg daily; pitavistatin starts at 2 mg and can be increased to 4 mg daily; rosuvastatin starts at 5 mg and other dosing intervals can include 10, 20, and 40 mg.

- Be aware that the doses of each of these medications are not equivalent in strength. For example, 10 mg of atorvastatin is felt to be the equivalent of 40 mg of pravastatin.

3 Do you know why are you being prescribed a statin medication?

☐ Heart disease

☐ High (>200 mg/dL) total cholesterol levels

☐ High (>200 mg/dL) triglyceride levels

☐ Recent heart attack

☐ Recent stroke or mini-stroke

☐ Family history of very high (>300 mg/dL) total cholesterol levels

☐ Other: _____

- If you are admitted to the hospital due to a heart attack or a stroke, part of the "pathways of care" for both of these diagnoses is treatment with a statin during your inpatient hospital stay. This is because statins have been demonstrated to improve overall life span and quality of life when given in these acute situations.

* * *

DOCTOR'S SPOTLIGHT

How Does Your Doctor Determine If You Need a Statin?

In the absence of a family history of really high cholesterol levels (which is an automatic yes to statin therapy), your doctor has a couple of assessment tools at his or her disposal for evaluating cardiovascular risk. One assessment tool from the American Heart Association/American College of Cardiology (AHA/ACC), based on recent findings from various studies, can be found at www.heart.org. Another risk stratification tool is something called a "Framingham risk score," which determines your risk of experiencing a heart attack within ten years, based on the following parameters:

- *Gender:* Men have a slightly increased risk of heart disease.
- *Age:* Risk of heart disease increases with age, beginning at forty-five.
- *Total cholesterol level:* Above 200 mg/dL confers a greater risk.
- *HDL cholesterol level:* Above 60 mg/dL is considered heart protective.
- *Systolic blood pressure:* There have been ongoing discussions, especially in light of recent clinical trials, about what the "goal blood pressure" should be, but most clinicians will agree a systolic blood pressure above 140–150 requires treatment.
- *Smoking history:* Smokers have an increased risk of heart disease, along with an increased risk of many other medical conditions, including cancer.

Numbers assigned to each parameter add up to a composite score used to determine your cardiac risk (i.e., your risk of developing heart disease over the next decade), which helps doctors to determine whether or not you need to be on a statin. There is a concern on the part of some clinicians as to whether or not this exaggerates true cardiac risk. See the Resources section in this book for links to the Framingham risk score and other guidelines that health professionals may use to assess cardiac risk and guide statin therapy.

* * *

4 Have you experienced any of the following symptoms while taking this medication?

☐ Unexplained pain in your muscles or joints

☐ Difficulty walking because of pain or fatigue

☐ Increased fatigue

☐ Problems with memory

☐ Blood in the urine [see next question]

☐ Other: _____

- Several studies have demonstrated that statin medications may be a cause of memory problems, though the association between memory loss and statin use has not been completely confirmed.

- Statin medications are known to cause muscle pain (myalgia or myopathy) and joint pain (arthralgia), which can sometimes be so debilitating that they can affect how you walk. Not everyone who takes statin medications will develop pain, however. For some individuals, switching from one statin medication to another can eliminate pain. Other individuals may not be tolerant of any of the medications in this class.

Coenzyme Q_{10}

A deficiency in coenzyme Q_{10}, also known as ubiquinone, may be a cause of statin-related myopathy. If a patient is being started on a statin, given that it can cause this deficiency, I often consider starting someone on a coenzyme Q_{10} supplement at the same time. Some studies suggest that this supplement may help decrease the intensity and frequency of statin-induced myopathy. Starting doses can be 50–100 mg daily, and this can be increased in frequency to two to three times a day. Check with your doctor to see if taking coenzyme Q_{10} is a good option for you if you suffer from statin-induced muscle or joint pain, and please refer to chapter 10 for more information on this supplement.

* * *

5 What blood tests are being used to monitor your medication?

☐ Liver function tests (AST and ALT levels)

☐ Creatinine levels

☐ Creatinine phosphokinase (CPK) levels

- With statin medications, your doctor should obtain blood work on a routine basis to ensure that the medication dosage you are taking is safe and does not require further adjustment.

- Because statin medications can affect your liver, it is recommended that liver tests be measured at the initiation of treatment and repeated if necessary.

- Doctors will routinely measure CPK levels in the blood, as elevated levels (another side effect of stain medications) may be a sign of damage to your muscles. *Note that some people can have muscle pain and normal CPK levels. Others can have increased CPK levels and little pain.* It is important that you pay attention to your lab work and symptoms to determine if you need to speak with your doctor to reduce or possibly discontinue your medication.

Rhabdomyolysis

Rhabdomyolysis refers to rapid muscle breakdown, which can be caused by statin medications. This can be indicated by a significant elevation in CPK levels or blood in the urine. Unrecognized and untreated rhabdomyolysis can cause acute injury to the kidneys. *If you see blood in your urine or notice that your urine is tea colored while taking a statin medication, please stop the medication and call your doctor immediately.*

* * *

6 Are you taking any of the following medications that might interact with statins?

☐ Lipid-lowering fibrates such as fenofibrate (TriCor) or gemfibrozil (Lopid)

☐ Niacin

☐ Calcium channel blockers such as diltiazem (Cardizem) and verapamil (Calan)

☐ Cyclosporine

☐ Macrolide antibiotics such as erythromycin (Erythrocin®) or clarithromycin (Biaxin®)

☐ Antifungal medications such as itraconazole (Sporanox®) and ketoconazole (Nizoral®)

- The combination of fibrates with a statin medication can increase the risk of developing the side effects of myalgia and worsening liver function. They can also increase the risk of developing rhabdomyolysis.

- Niacin is prescribed by physicians to increase HDL levels if they are low. Examples of prescription formulations include Niaspan® (an extended-release tablet). Niacin also can be purchased in supplement form over the counter. As with fibrates, the combination of niacin with a statin medication can also increase the risk of developing myalgia and worsening liver function.

- The calcium channel blockers noted above, antifungal medications, and cyclosporine can inhibit the metabolism of statins in the liver.

This can increase the *half-life* (the time it takes for 50 percent of the medication to be eliminated from your body) of these medications in the blood, which also increases the risk of developing side effects.

- Simvastatin (Zocor) and atorvastatin (Lipitor) are primarily metabolized by CYP3A4 in the liver. Why does this matter? Because macrolide antibiotics such as erythromycin and clarithromycin are processed by the same pathway, and they can inhibit the metabolism of simvastatin and atorvastatin. The longer simvastatin, lovastatin, and atorvastatin stay in the system, the higher the chance of developing side effects.

THE PERSONALIZED APPROACH
Combining Statin Therapy with Other Drugs

The following example demonstrates how knowledge of drug metabolism pathways combined with personalized blood testing can help doctors determine the appropriate medications and dosages, while potentially minimizing the risk of developing side effects and harmful interactions.

Mrs. X is an elderly female with a history of high blood pressure, gout, reflux, and chronic kidney disease. Her medications included metoprolol (a beta blocker), Zocor (a statin), and tramadol (Ultram®, a narcotic-like pain medication). Given that her kidney function was abnormal, we decided to keep her on a very low, 10-mg daily dosage of Zocor, which is metabolized by the cytochrome 3A4 pathway in the liver. If her pharmacokinetic profile had shown that she was a poor metabolizer of the cytochrome 3A4 pathway, we would not have chosen Zocor for her.

Her blood pressure was controlled for most of the day, but she noted that it would sometimes decrease later in the evening. She also reported having arthritis pain that was not completely relieved with her current pain medication. The results of her personalized testing confirmed what her lower blood pressure at night suggested: She was an "intermediate metabolizer" of metoprolol, meaning that this medication stays in her bloodstream longer than average. Her dose of metoprolol was subsequently decreased by half. Testing also confirmed that she was an intermediate metabolizer of Ultram, so increasing the frequency of this medication was not an option, and given that she was a poor metabolizer of the 3A5 pathway, other pain medications such as fentanyl (processed in the liver by this particular pathway) were not good choices.

Thus, we elected to start the patient on turmeric—an orange spice found in many Indian dishes and believed to have anti-inflammatory effects—and reduce her statin dose if the pain continued.

If someone is a slow "metabolizer" of a particular pathway, the use of a medication processed by that particular pathway would be discouraged. If there were no substitute medication, a very low dose would be considered (and very slowly increased, if needed), and he or she would be closely monitored for side effects. If a medication is known to inhibit a certain pathway, and the patient is a slow metabolizer of that pathway, prescribing that medication is a double no-no. In the above example, let's say Mrs. X was dealing with a bout of acute bacterial bronchitis, and her physician wanted her to be on clarithromycin (Biaxin). If she is on Zocor and is a poor metabolizer to begin with, then putting her on a medication like Biaxin, which can inhibit the CYP3A4 pathway, will doubly increase her chances of developing a medication reaction. The use of another antibiotic, such as azithromycin (Zithromax®), which would inhibit this pathway only minimally, would be a reasonable alternative. Hence, this example shows how the use of testing to personalize medication regimens can decrease the risk of developing serious side effects.

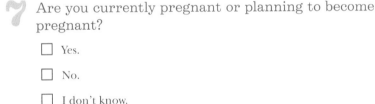

Are you currently pregnant or planning to become pregnant?

☐ Yes.

☐ No.

☐ I don't know.

- While there is ongoing debate among health professionals concerning how dangerous statins may be to the developing fetus, it is still recommended that these medications be avoided if you are pregnant or planning to become pregnant.

Ezetimibe (Zetia)

While statin therapies work by inhibiting the production of cholesterol, Zetia works by blocking the absorption of cholesterol in the intestine. This medication can be used alone for the treatment of high cholesterol levels, but doctors most commonly prescribe Zetia when patients do not tolerate statin therapy or if statin therapy is not enough to decrease the cholesterol to healthy levels. In many cases, statins and Zetia can be taken together, and they are an effective combination.

1 Are you currently taking Zetia?

☐ Yes.

☐ No.

- The dosing of Zetia is easy to remember: 10 mg, taken once daily.

2 Have you experienced any of the following symptoms while taking this medication?

☐ Skin rash

☐ Abdominal or back pain

☐ Joint pain (arthralgia)

☐ Muscle pain (myalgia)

☐ Jaundice

☐ Fever

☐ Other: _____

- There have been case reports of Zetia causing myalgia when taken on its own.

- While there have been some case reports of mild increases in liver enzymes when Zetia is taken on its own, this effect is uncommon. Nevertheless, we do recommend that you have your liver function tested regularly.

- *Zetia can cause a skin rash. If this occurs, stop taking the medication and call your physician, as you may be having an allergic reaction.*

- *This medication has also been reported to cause fever, abdominal pain, and jaundice (yellowing of the skin) in some people. If you experience any of these symptoms, stop the medication and call your doctor immediately.* Jaundice is an especially serious side effect that may indicate an acute problem with the liver.

3 Are you taking any of the following medications that might interact with Zetia?

☐ Statins

☐ Fibrates such as fenofibrate (TriCor) or gemfibrozil (Lopid)

☐ Bile acid sequestrants such as cholestyramine

- While statins and Zetia are commonly taken together, there is a risk of developing elevated liver enzymes and myopathy. Your doctor will need to monitor your blood work, including your liver function and CPK levels.

- When fibrates are taken in conjunction with Zetia, your liver function should be monitored as well. If you develop any muscle or joint pain with this combination, let your doctor know, and a CPK test will be ordered.

- Because they work in a similar fashion—by blocking the absorption of cholesterol in the intestines—taking both Zetia and a bile acid sequestrant at the same time can affect each medication's ability to work at maximum efficiency. They need to be taken five to six hours apart from each other. If you are taking Zetia at night, for example, it may be a good idea to take cholestyramine in the morning.

Bile Acid Sequestrants

These medications lower your cholesterol levels by blocking the absorption of cholesterol in the small intestine. One bile acid sequestrant, colesevelam (Welchol®), is also prescribed for the treatment of diabetes because it helps lower blood glucose levels. These medications can be taken in conjunction with statin medications and Zetia.

1 Which (if any) of the following bile acid sequestrants are you currently taking?

☐ Colesevelam (Welchol)

☐ Colestipol (Colestid®)

☐ Cholestyramine (LoCholest®)

☐ Other: _____

2 What dose are you currently taking, at what frequency?

_____ mg _____ times a day.

- Be sure that you take Zetia several hours after taking any of the bile acid sequestrants. Taking these medications close together can decrease the efficacy of Zetia.

- Colesevelam (Welchol) comes in both pill form and packet form. If you have the pill form, take it during meals. You can either take all six pills with one meal, or you can take half the doses with your two largest meals of the day. If you have the packet form, you must prepare and drink the liquid during meals.

- Colestipol (Colestid) can be taken once or twice a day with meals.

- Cholestyramine (LoCholest) is usually prescribed in powdered form, to be taken in doses of 4 grams, one to three times a day before meals.

3 Have you experienced any of the following symptoms while taking this medication?

☐ Acid reflux

☐ Loose stools

☐ Constipation

☐ Abdominal discomfort

☐ Difficulties with digestion

☐ Gallstones

☐ Other: _____

- Bile acid sequestrants are designed to stay in the gut, so side effects are usually confined to the gastrointestinal tract. If these symptoms persist for a few days after starting any of these medications, please call your doctor.

- The incidence of gallstones is increased, especially if bile acid seques-trants are taken concomitantly with ezetimibe (Zetia).

4 Are you currently taking any of the following medications or supplements that might interact with bile acid sequestrants?

☐ Iron supplements

☐ Vitamins A, D, E, and/or K

☐ Thyroid medications such as levothyroxine or Armour® Thyroid tablets

☐ Warfarin

☐ Digoxin (Lanoxin)

☐ Statin medications

- In addition to preventing the reabsorption of bile into the gut, bile acid sequestrants can also prevent the absorption of other medications and supplements. The substances listed above especially need to be taken several hours apart from bile acid sequestrants.

- *It is important that you take your iron supplements and your thyroid medication separate from ALL of your other medications*—not just bile acid sequestrants. *Iron and thyroid medication should also be taken separately from each other by a couple of hours.* Allow thirty minutes to one hour for these substances to be absorbed by your intestine.

- This class of medications can also affect the absorption of fat-soluble vitamins. This includes vitamins A, D, E, and K. If you are taking bile acid sequestrants, talk with your doctor about how to supplement with these vitamins, and please see chapter 10.

- Given the effect that this class of medications has on the absorption of vitamin K, if you are on warfarin, your blood concentration levels of this drug need to be monitored closely. Please see chapter 7 for more information on warfarin and its many significant drug interactions.

PCSK9 Inhibitors

These are the newest class of cholesterol-lowering medications. They target the LDL receptor, helping to decrease the circulating LDL levels. These medications are prescribed for the treatment of certain genetic conditions associated with high cholesterol levels, but they are also prescribed for patients whose LDL cholesterol levels are difficult to lower with the other medications in this chapter.

1 Which (if any) of the following PCSK9 inhibitors are you currently taking?

☐ Alirocumab (Praluent®)

☐ Evolocumab (Repatha™)

☐ Other: _____

2 What dose are you currently taking, at what frequency?

_____ mg _____ times a month.

- Alirocumab (Praluent) is not prescribed in pill form, but rather given as an injection under the skin (subcutaneous) every two weeks. The initial dose is 75 mg, and, depending on your blood work, it can be increased to 150 mg.

- Evolocumab (Repatha) is also given as an injection; the initial dose is 140 mg, twice weekly. Once-a-month dosing is available as well.

3 Have you experienced any of the following symptoms while taking this medication?

☐ Tiredness

☐ Weakness

☐ Muscle aches (myalgia)

☐ Joint aches and pains (arthralgia)

☐ Confusion

☐ Other: _____

- If you are experiencing any of these reactions, please call your physician or health-care provider.

Fibrates

This medication class is prescribed for the treatment of high triglyceride levels (e.g., greater than 150–200 mg/dL) when they cannot be lowered through diet and exercise.

1 Which (if any) of the following medications are you currently taking?

☐ Gemfibrozil (Lopid)

☐ Fenofibrate (TriCor)

☐ Other: _____

2 What dose are you currently taking, at what frequency?

_____ mg _____ times a day.

- Gemfibrozil (Lopid) is usually prescribed at 600 mg, twice a day.
- Fenofibrate (TriCor) comes in two different dosages: 48 mg and 148 mg. Both are taken once a day.

3 Have you experienced any of the following symptoms while taking this medication?

☐ Unexplained pain in your muscles or joints

☐ Increased fatigue

☐ Difficulty walking because of pain or fatigue

☐ Blood in the urine

☐ Gallstones

☐ Other: _____

- Much of what you read concerning statin medications also holds true for fibrates. *They can cause myopathy, fatigue, and even rhabdomyolysis. If you are experiencing any of these side effects, do not hesitate to call your doctor.*

- Fibrates can also increase the risk of developing gallstones.

4 Are you taking any of the following medications that might interact with fibrates?

☐ Statins

☐ Ezetimibe (Zetia)

☐ Any other fibrates

- The combination of fibrates with statin or other fibrate medications, with or without Zetia, can increase the risk of developing increased liver AST or ALT levels, as well as myopathy. If you are on these medications, or a combination of these medications, your doctor should be monitoring you closely.

* * *

SUPPLEMENT SPOTLIGHT

Fish Oil

Fish oil is a natural supplement that can be obtained over the counter or in prescription form for a variety of purposes. Vascepa® is a synthetic derivative of fish oil prescribed by physicians for treating elevated triglyceride levels. It has high antioxidant properties and doses start at 3–4 grams a day. Lovaza® is another prescription-strength omega-3 fish oil that is used for the same purpose. Starting at doses of 1–2 grams per day, this supplement can be taken in conjunction with fibrates. For more information on this supplement, please see chapter 10 and speak with your doctor.

* * *

Notes

Notes

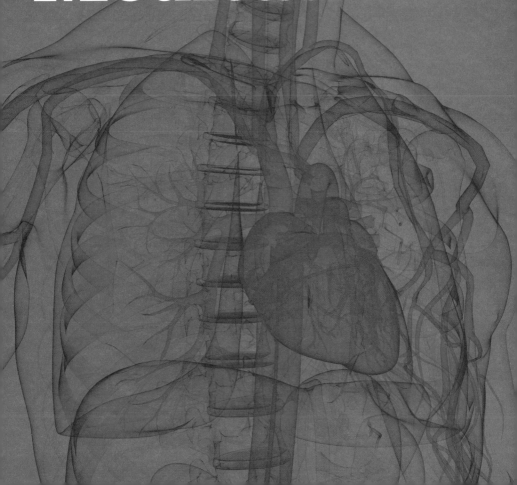

Heart
& Blood
Pressure
Medications

Heart & Blood Pressure Medications

HEART DISEASE AND CHRONIC HEART FAILURE (CHF) REMAIN THE most common reasons for patients to be admitted to the hospital. High blood pressure is a condition that affects millions of Americans and, along with diabetes, is a leading risk factor for the development of heart disease. This chapter reviews the many types of blood pressure–lowering (antihypertensive) medications. One important aspect of many of these medications is their versatility: not only do they have blood pressure–lowering effects, but many have other heart-protective effects as well.

Angiotensin-converting enzyme inhibitors (**ACE inhibitors**, for short) are one of the most common medications prescribed by physicians. In addition to being effective for lowering blood pressure, they have heart- and kidney-protective effects. Commonly prescribed medications in this class include lisinopril (Zestril®), enalapril (Vasotec®), and ramipril (Altace®). One of the main possible side effects of ACE inhibitors is high potassium (hyperkalemia).

Many clinicians will prescribe **angiotensin receptor blockers (ARBs)** if patients are intolerant to ACE inhibitors, though the two classes are closely related. Like ACE inhibitors, these medications can also cause high potassium levels that need to be monitored. Commonly prescribed medications in this class include valsartan (Diovan®), losartan (Cozaar®), and olmesartan (Benicar®).

Calcium channel blockers (CCBs) are used to treat high blood pressure, but certain medications in this class are also used for the treatment of abnormal heart rhythms (arrhythmias). They have kidney-protective effects and stroke-preventive properties as well. Commonly prescribed medications in this class include amlodipine (Norvasc®), felodipine (Plendil®), verapamil (Calan), and diltiazem (Cardizem®).

Beta blockers provide significant protection for the heart. They are commonly prescribed after a heart attack and also for the treatment of CHF. Studies have shown that they can extend the life span of those who have either (or both) of these conditions. Commonly prescribed medications in this class include metoprolol (Lopressor®), atenolol (Tenormin®), carvedilol (Coreg®), and nadolol (Corgard®).

Diuretics may be prescribed solely for the treatment of high blood pressure or in combination with other medications described above. Certain diuretics can also be used for the treatment of CHF as well as swelling (edema). Possible side effects of this class of medications include dehydration and low potassium and magnesium levels. If you are taking any diuretics, it is extremely important that you pay close attention to this section, as there are nuances with these medications of which you need to be aware. Commonly prescribed medications include hydrochlorothiazide (HCTZ), chlorthalidone (Hygroton®), furosemide (Lasix®), and torsemide (Demadex®).

Potassium-sparing diuretics are commonly prescribed for the treatment of CHF and high blood pressure. Medications in this class include spironolactone (Aldactone), eplerenone (Inspra), and amiloride (Midamor®). Studies have demonstrated that Aldactone and Inspra can be very effective for the treatment of high blood pressure that is otherwise difficult to treat (a.k.a. resistant hypertension).

Other medication classes prescribed for the treatment of blood pressure include **alpha blockers** and the centrally acting agent **clonidine** (Catapres®). **Nitrates** are used for the treatment of angina (chest pain) as well as acute and chronic CHF.

* * *

CONDITION SPOTLIGHT

Chronic Heart Failure

Chronic heart failure (often called "congestive heart failure") is the leading reason that individuals are not only admitted to the hospital but also readmitted within a thirty-day timeframe. There are basically two different types of CHF: Heart failure with reduced ejection fraction (HFrEF, a.k.a. "systolic heart failure") refers to an inability of the heart to pump the blood as effectively as it is supposed to, and heart failure with preserved ejection fraction (HFpEF, a.k.a. "diastolic heart failure") refers to an inability of the heart to "relax." The latter is more common than the former, although both may be present in the same individual. High blood pressure and heart disease are risk factors for the development of CHF, and diabetes and kidney disease are often present as comorbidities in patients who have been diagnosed with the condition.

If you have been diagnosed with HFrEF, medications that you will likely be prescribed include beta blockers, loop diuretics (to manage edema and shortness of breath), and a medication called digoxin (Lanoxin), which helps improve the symptoms of heart failure. ACE inhibitors or ARBs will likely also be prescribed to help "remodel" the heart or restore normal heart-pump function. You may also be prescribed a potassium-sparing diuretic such as spironolactone (Aldactone) or medications such as isosorbide dinitrate (Isordil®) and hydralazine (Apresoline®).

If you have been diagnosed with HFpEF, ACE inhibitors and ARBs are not as beneficial as beta blockers and/or calcium channel blockers, which are typically prescribed to help the "stiff" heart to "relax" better. Preventing the blood pressure from getting too high is also important when a patient has diastolic CHF.

If you have been diagnosed with either type of CHF, it is important that you do the following:

- Weigh yourself daily and record your weights. If you are on a diuretic, you need to examine the trend, as fluid can be gained and lost each day. My standing rule of thumb is that if a person's weight increases by two pounds in two consecutive days, then his or her diuretic dosage needs to be modified upward.
- The converse of this is also true. If you are losing more than two pounds in two days, then you should call your doctor about reducing your diuretic dosage.
- Your doctor will talk with you about the importance of being on a fluid restriction of about a quart to a quart and a half a day.
- Studies demonstrate that a modest sodium restriction is important for minimizing fluid-related weight gain. In a hospital setting, most individuals with CHF will be placed on a sodium restriction of 2 grams per day. This means that at home a sodium restriction of 2,000–2,250 mg is reasonable. Many people who had high sodium diets will not tolerate a drastic reduction in their sodium intake, and recent studies are making doctors rethink the benefits versus the risks of severe sodium restriction.
- Following a plant-based diet, such as the Dietary Approaches to Stop Hypertension (DASH) diet or the healthy and much touted Mediterranean diet can really benefit the heart. It can be challenging for people to adopt a strict plant-based diet, although many do. In my experience, people prefer the Mediterranean diet because it is very flexible and offers significant variety.
- Check with your doctor to see if you can exercise on a daily basis. Even walking on five to ten minutes a day at a steady pace provides cardiovascular benefits.
- Your blood work—including potassium, magnesium, and creatinine levels—should be monitored closely, especially if there is an increase in the dosing of the ACE inhibitor, ARB, or any of the diuretics.
- In addition to tracking your weight at home, regularly checking your blood pressure and pulse rate is important. *If you find your blood pressure is getting really low, especially if you are feeling dizzy and lightheaded, then don't hesitate to call your doctor.*
- If you have nausea, vomiting, or diarrhea for longer than a few hours, then call your doctor to see if you should stop taking your ACE inhibitor, diuretic, and/or ARB. These medications can make kidney function worse, and taking the diuretic may also increase your risk of dehydration.
- *If you notice a decrease in the amount that you are urinating, please call your doctor.* This can mean many things, but a doctor might wonder if this is a sign of dehydration or worsening kidney function.

* * *

Angiotensin-Converting Enzyme (ACE) Inhibitors

If you have HFeEF, the heart does not squeeze as well as it should. This class of medications inhibits an enzyme that causes the heart muscles to contract, allowing the blood vessels to dilate, which can make it easier for your heart to pump blood and can really help improve your heart function over time. ACE inhibitors are also a preferred class of medications for the treatment of high blood pressure. If your doctor wants to prescribe an ACE inhibitor, you should go through this checklist before beginning on the new drug.

1 Which (if any) of the following ACE inhibitors are you currently taking?

☐ Ramipril (Altace)

☐ Lisinopril (Zestril)

☐ Enalapril (Vasotec)

☐ Fosinopril (Monopril®)

☐ Quinapril (Accupril®)

☐ Other: _____

- If your doctor wants to prescribe an ACE inhibitor or you checked off more than one medication in this list, please talk to your doctor right away. Taking more than one type of ACE inhibitor will increase the risk of developing side effects. It may raise your potassium levels dangerously high and has the potential to worsen your kidney function.

 What dose are you currently taking, at what frequency?

_____ mg _____ times a day.

- Enalapril (Vasotec) can be dosed 5 or 10 mg, once or twice a day.

- Lisinopril (Zestril) can be started at 2.5 mg or 5 mg and dosed once a day.

- Ramipril (Altace) is often started at doses of 2.5–5 mg and can be taken once or twice a day.

- The dose range for fosinopril (Monopril) and quinapril (Accupril) is 10, 20, and 40 mg, once or twice a day.

3 Why have you been prescribed this medication?

☐ High blood pressure

☐ Recent or previous heart attack

☐ CHF

☐ Leaking of protein in the urine due to diabetes (proteinuria)

☐ Other: _____

- The above medical conditions represent the most common reasons why your doctor may have prescribed an ACE inhibitor. Diabetes, high blood pressure, and CHF often occur together.

4 Have you experienced any of the following symptoms while taking this medication?

☐ Cough

☐ Swelling of the throat and/or tongue (angioedema)

☐ Dizziness or lightheadedness

☐ Other: _____

- One of the major side effects of blood pressure–lowering medications is dizziness or lightheadedness, especially after standing up. Do your best to avoid sudden movements and try sitting upright before standing up.

- Another common side effect is a nagging, nonproductive cough that doesn't seem to go away. This can occur even after taking this medication for several months. If the cough is persistent and frequent, your doctor may recommend that you stop the medication to see if it goes away. If it does, you may need to try a different drug to avoid this side effect.

- An infrequent, but VERY SERIOUS side effect of this medication is swelling of the throat or tongue (angioedema). *If you think you are experiencing this, call 911 immediately and stop taking the medication.*

5 Have you had blood work done to evaluate your potassium levels or kidney function?

☐ Yes.

☐ No.

- If you have been started on this medication, ask your doctor if you should be given blood work to have your kidney function and potassium level checked.

6 Are you taking any of the following medications that might interact with ACE inhibitors?

☐ Nonsteroidal anti-inflammatory drugs (NSAIDs) such as ibuprofen or naproxen (Aleve®)

☐ Angiotensin receptor blockers

☐ Diuretics such as spironolactone (Aldactone), eplerenone (Inspra), or furosemide (Lasix)

☐ Sulfamethoxazole/trimethoprim (Bactrim)

- ACE inhibitors can worsen kidney function and raise potassium levels in some individuals. This risk increases if you are dehydrated or if you are taking ACE inhibitors in addition to one or more of the following classes of medications: ARBs, potassium-sparing diuretics, and NSAIDs. For more information on NSAIDs and other pain medications, please refer to chapter 8.

- Note that the combination of ACE inhibitors and potassium-sparing diuretics such as spironolactone (Aldactone) has very beneficial effects on the heart and kidneys, and many individuals on both of these medications do fine. It is when the body gets out of balance because of an acute illness—viral gastroenteritis, dehydration, etc.—that this medication combination can be harmful. I advise CHF patients to call me if an acute illness occurs so that I can temporarily hold or adjust the dosage of these medications. In this situation, I would also check blood work and follow their daily weight and symptoms closely. In many cases, these medications can be continued after the acute illness resolves.

- Bactrim is an antibiotic that can raise potassium levels. See chapter 9 for more information on this.

- *If you are taking NSAIDs, ACE inhibitors, ARBs, diuretics, and/or Bactrim either alone or in combination, your kidney function and potassium levels should be monitored periodically. If you develop nausea, vomiting, diarrhea, or any acute illness while on these medications—especially if you are taking them in combination with one another—call your doctor immediately, as some or all of these drugs may need to be temporarily discontinued until you recover.*

Why Do We Care About Potassium Levels?

Your heart is an electrical circuit. Potassium levels (normally 3.5 to 5 millimoles per liter [mmol/L]) that are too high or too low can potentially disrupt this circuitry. If your potassium levels are really high, say 5.7 mmol/L or greater, this can slow your heart rate and rhythm down. If your potassium is on the really low side, 3.0 mmol/L or less, this can increase the "irritability" of the heart and also may increase the risk of developing an arrhythmia in some individuals. While many arrhythmias are not serious, some can result in cardiac arrest. Note that if you are on an ACE inhibitor together with an ARB, you are at a significantly increased risk of developing high potassium levels, in addition to compromised kidney function.

* * *

Angiotensin Receptor Blockers (ARBs)

ARBs have many of the same indications as ACE inhibitors, including the treatment of high blood pressure, CHF, heart attack, and proteinuria, but this class does not produce the persistent cough that ACE inhibitors sometimes do. While ARBs can cause high potassium levels, this side effect may be less severe than that of ACE inhibitors.

1 Which (if any) of the following ARBs are you currently taking?

☐ Valsartan (Diovan)

☐ Olmesartan (Benicar)

☐ Telmisartan (Micardis®)

☐ Losartan (Cozaar)

☐ Candesartan (Atacand®)

☐ Other: _____

2 What dose are you currently taking, at what frequency?

_____ mg _____ times a day

- Valsartan (Diovan) can be dosed as low as 40 mg and as high as 320 mg daily, or in divided doses twice a day.

- Olmesartan (Benicar) can be started as low as 5 mg to as high as 40 mg, once a day.

- Telmisartan (Micardis) is usually dosed 40 or 80 mg, once a day.

- Losartan (Cozaar) can be dosed 25–100 mg, once or twice a day.

- Candesartan (Atacand) is usually dosed 4–32 mg, to be taken once a day.

3 Why have you been prescribed this medication?

☐ High blood pressure

☐ Recent or previous heart attack

☐ CHF

☐ Leaking of protein in the urine due to diabetes (proteinuria)

☐ Other: _____

4 Have you experienced any of the following symptoms while taking this medication?

☐ Nausea

☐ Stomach upset

☐ Dizziness

☐ Skin rash

☐ Angioedema

☐ Other: _____

- As with any blood pressure medication, common symptoms are nausea, stomach upset, dizziness, and/or rash. If these symptoms persist for a few days, stop taking this medication and call your doctor.

- *If you were prescribed an ARB because you were on an ACE inhibitor that caused angioedema, it is important to keep in mind that, in some individuals, certain ARBs may potentially cause angioedema as well.* If you have been on an ACE inhibitor and are switching over to an ARB because of this reaction, it is a good idea to have this discussion with your doctor.

5 Are you taking any of the following medications that might interact with ARBs?

☐ Nonsteroidal anti-inflammatory drugs (NSAIDs) such as ibuprofen or naproxen (Aleve)

☐ An ACE inhibitor

☐ Diuretics including hydrochlorothiazide (HCTZ), furosemide (Lasix), or spironolactone (Aldactone)

☐ Sulfamethoxazole/trimethoprim (Bactrim)

- Like ACE inhibitors, ARBs can worsen kidney function and raise potassium levels in some individuals. This risk increases if you are taking ARBs in addition to the following classes of medications: ACE inhibitors, diuretics (especially potassium-sparing diuretics), and NSAIDs.

- *If you taking ARBs in addition to NSAIDs and/or other medications listed above and develop nausea, vomiting, diarrhea, or any acute illness, call your doctor immediately.*

Calcium Channel Blockers (CCBs)

CCBs are one of the first-line therapies for blood pressure control. These are commonly combined with ACE inhibitors, ARBs, and/or diuretics to have a synergistic effect on lowering blood pressure.

1 Which (if any) of the following CCBs are you currently taking?

☐ Amlodipine (Norvasc)

☐ Felodipine (Plendil)

☐ Nifedipine XL (Procardia®)

☐ Diltiazem (Cardizem)

☐ Verapamil (Calan)

☐ Other: _____

- There are two broad categories of CCBs. The first category, known as "vasodilators," works to lower blood pressure by dilating the blood vessels. Medications in this category include amlodipine (Norvasc), felodipine (Plendil), and nifedipine (Procardia).

- Verapamil (Calan) and diltiazem (Cardizem) belong to a second category that works by normalizing heart rhythm and lowering the heart rate when the heart beats too fast. They are often prescribed for heart rhythm abnormalities. These CCBs would be a good option for someone who has both hypertension and tachycardia (abnormally fast heartbeat). They have some vasodilator properties as well.

2 What dose are you currently taking, at what frequency?

_____ mg _____ times a day.

- Amlodipine (Norvasc) is a once-a-day medication. Dose ranges include 2.5, 5, and 10 mg.

- Felodipine (Plendil) can be taken once or twice a day at doses of 5–10 mg.

- Nifedipine (Procardia XL) doses range from 30 to 120 mg, taken daily.

- There are different formulations of diltiazem (Cardizem), and the short-acting formulation can be taken several times a day. For example, if someone has an abnormal heart rhythm, the cardiologist will sometimes prescribe this medication to be taken three to four times a day and then switch the patient to a longer-acting, once-a-day formulation when his or her heart rhythm stabilizes and the doctor can determine how much will be needed over a twenty-four-hour period.

- Verapamil (Calan) is often prescribed to be taken two to four times a day. There is also a sustained-release formulation for once-a-day dosing.

3 Why have you been prescribed this medication?

☐ High blood pressure

☐ CHF

☐ Treatment of abnormal heart rhythms

☐ Blood circulation problems (Raynaud's phenomenon)

☐ Other: _____

- Many physicians will prescribe this class of medications for patients who are not able to tolerate beta blockers. Examples of why you may not be able to tolerate beta blockers include acute asthma and poorly controlled diabetes.

- Verapamil (Calan) and diltiazem (Cardizem) are prescribed for cardiac arrhythmia, and the most common type of arrhythmia they are used to treat is atrial fibrillation. They also can help to reduce blood pressure but may not be as effective as other CCBs for this purpose. They are also used for the treatment of Raynaud's phenomenon to help improve blood circulation.

What Should Be Your Blood Pressure Goal?

What exactly is the goal range for blood pressure? While there are guidelines, they have been a matter of much debate among health-care professionals. Here is the argument in a nutshell: An organization called the Joint National Committee 8 came together in December 2013 and not only made recommendations in terms of first-line treatment for high blood pressure (ACE inhibitors, ARBs, diuretics, and/or CCBs), but also what the range of goal blood pressures should be. These guidelines actually raised the goal ranges for blood pressure, compared with preceding guidelines.

- If you are a healthy person with no other health problems, and you are less than sixty years of age, your blood pressure goal should be 140/90 mmHg or less.
- If you are older than sixty, your blood pressure goal should have 150/90 mmHg as an upper limit.
- If you have diabetes and/or kidney disease, your blood pressure should be less than 140/90 mmHg.

It is important to understand that many clinical trials evaluating the effectiveness of blood pressure–lowering treatments noted a significant risk reduction in events such as heart attack and stroke in individuals under sixty years of age, but no additional benefit was noted for individuals over eighty years of age. Because patients between ages sixty and eighty are underrepresented in the clinical trials, this committee applied the 150/90 guideline to ages sixty and up, however.

To their credit, the experts are trying to "personalize" the blood pressure goals based on challenges associated with the age and general health of the patient. For example, if you are an older person with a history of high blood pressure that has been difficult to control for many years, your blood pressure goal should not be as low as 120/80 mmHg. Making your blood pressure goal too low increases your risk of dizziness as well as your fall risk. In the elderly, this is a significant concern.

Bottom line: You and your doctor should engage in shared decision-making concerning your blood pressure goals. Depending on your risk factors, concerns, and prior responses to medications, this is the best way to establish realistic and reachable goals.

* * *

4 Have you experienced any of the following symptoms while taking your CCB?

☐ Fatigue

☐ Headaches

☐ Heartburn

☐ Swelling of the ankles or feet (edema)

☐ Flushing of the skin

☐ Constipation

☐ Dizziness

☐ Difficulty breathing or wheezing

☐ Other: _____

- This class of medications is tolerated well by most patients, but the major common side effects we see in clinical practice include constipation and edema. The use of a stool softener may be recommended if you cannot be switched to another medication. If there is significant swelling, the dosage may need to be decreased or discontinued. The use of a diuretic such as furosemide (Lasix) may be prescribed to help control edema.

- Your body's way of cooling off requires the dilation of your blood vessels, so you may notice that your legs "swell" more in the summer while on a CCB. The excessive use of a diuretic to combat this side effect can increase the risk of developing dehydration. Please speak with your doctor if you find this occurring.

- *If you develop difficulty breathing, stop taking the medication and call 911.*

5 Are you currently taking any of the following medications that might interact with CCBs?

☐ Beta blockers

☐ Amiodarone (Cordarone) (an antiarrhythmic)

☐ Digoxin (Lanoxin)

☐ Sotalol (Betapace®) (a nonselective beta blocker)

☐ Macrolide antibiotics such as erythromycin or clarithromycin (Biaxin)

☐ Any other class of heart and blood pressure medications discussed in this chapter

- Combining verapamil (Calan) or diltiazem (Cardizem) with any of the above medications may cause hypotension (low blood pressure) or bradycardia (slow heart rate).

- Amlodipine (Norvasc) may be prescribed by your doctor for better blood pressure control and to avoid potential risk of bradycardia.

- Because many CCBs are metabolized by the CYP3A4 pathway, the use of certain macrolide antibiotics may inhibit their metabolism, which could increase the risk of developing low blood pressure, or hypotension. This important interaction is discussed in chapter 9.

Beta Blockers

Beta blockers, also known as beta-adrenergic blocking agents, are medications that work by blocking the effects of the hormone epinephrine, also known as adrenaline. When you take beta blockers, your heart beats more slowly and with less force, thereby reducing blood pressure. They also help blood vessels open up to improve blood flow.

1 Why are you being prescribed a beta blocker?

☐ Heart attack

☐ CHF

☐ High blood pressure

☐ Essential tremors

☐ Migraines

☐ Palpitations

☐ Atrial fibrillation or other abnormal heart rhythms

☐ Other: _____

- One of the primary reasons beta blockers are prescribed is that they have been shown to improve morbidity and mortality in patients suffering from an acute heart attack and/or CHF.

- While they may reduce blood pressure, this is not what they are primarily used for.

- Beta blockers are also prescribed to prevent migraines and tremors.

- Other uses for beta blockers include the treatment of symptoms associated with hyperthyroidism and liver disease (cirrhosis).

2 **Which (if any) of the following beta blockers are you currently taking?**

☐ Metoprolol (Lopressor, Toprol-XL®)

☐ Nadolol (Corgard)

☐ Atenolol (Tenormin)

☐ Carvedilol (Coreg)

☐ Propanolol (Inderal)

☐ Bisoprolol (Zebeta®)

☐ Other: _____

- Certain types of beta blockers are better for certain conditions than others. For example, metoprolol (Lopressor, Toprol-XL), carvedilol (Coreg), and bisoprolol (Zebeta) are the three medications among all of the beta blockers preferred for the treatment of CHF.

- Propanolol (Inderal) is probably better than the other beta blockers for the treatment of essential tremors because, unlike the other medications, it can penetrate the blood-brain barrier.

- Nadolol (Corgard) has been prescribed for the treatment of cirrhosis and liver disease. It works by lowering portal venous pressures in the liver, which can help increase the life span of that organ.

....

THE PERSONALIZED APPROACH

The Pharmacogenetics of Metoprolol

Dr. Khalighi and his team have performed studies concerning the pharmacogenetics of metoprolol (Lopressor, Toprol-XL). Note that while this medication is metabolized and inactivated by the CYP2D6 pathway in the liver, there can be close to one hundred genetic variations of this pathway among different individuals. Some of these variations can affect the metabolism of metoprolol so that either it is degraded in your body at a lower-than-normal rate, resulting in increased side effects such as fatigue; or the medication may be inactivated at a faster-than-normal rate, leading to an inadequate effect.

After performing DNA sequencing analysis of the CYP2D6 gene in 304 patients, a subsequent analysis led to individualized metoprolol recommendations based on their CYP2D6 genotypes. Dr. Khalighi found that up to 60 percent of the tested patients had genetic variations that led to a sub-optimal effect of metoprolol. For poor-metabolizer patients, lowering the dose or switching to alternatives that are not metabolized by CYP2D6—such as atenolol (Tenormin) or nadolol (Corgard)—decreased major side effects, while increasing the dose of metoprolol for rapid-metabolizer patients increased the medication's efficacy.

....

3 Do you have liver or kidney disease?

☐ Yes.

☐ No.

☐ I don't know.

- Many beta blockers are processed by the liver, so dose adjustments might be required in the setting of reduced liver function.

- Atenolol (Tenormin) and nadolol (Corgard) are eliminated by the body via the kidneys, so if your kidney function is abnormal, then the dose of this medication may need to be reduced or another medication may need to be chosen.

* * *

MEDICATION SPOTLIGHT

Stopping Beta Blockers

Beta blockers cannot be stopped abruptly. The dose needs to be reduced slowly over a few weeks' time. If they are stopped abruptly, a withdrawal reaction may occur. In this situation, you could potentially experience very high blood pressure and a fast heart rate, which can be very serious. *Please do not stop any medication in this class without first speaking with your doctor.*

* * *

4 Have you experienced any of the following symptoms while taking this medication?

☐ Fatigue

☐ Depression

☐ Impotence or sexual dysfunction

☐ Dizziness or lightheadedness

☐ Slow heart rate (bradycardia)

☐ Low blood pressure (hypotension)

☐ Shortness of breath

☐ Wheezing

☐ Other: _____

- Beta blockers generally are not prescribed to people diagnosed with asthma because of concerns that the medication may trigger a severe asthma attack.

- If you have diabetes, beta blockers may block signs of low blood sugar, such as rapid heartbeat and hand tremor. It's important to monitor your blood sugar on a regular basis.

- If you are experiencing any of the above symptoms and you are on this class of medication, talk with your health-care provider to see if the medication may be contributing to your symptoms.

5 Are you taking any of the following medications that might interact with beta blockers?

☐ CCBs including verapamil (Calan) and diltiazem (Cardizem)

☐ Digoxin (Lanoxin)

☐ Amiodarone (Cordarone)

☐ Sotalol (Betapace)

☐ Clonidine (Catapres)

☐ Other blood pressure medications listed in this chapter

☐ Cholesterol-lowering fibrate medications including fenofibrate (TriCor) and gemfibrozil (Lopid)

☐ Cyclosporine (Neoral®)

☐ Anticonvulsants such as phenobarbital (Luminal®), phenytoin (Dilantin), and carbamazepine (Tegretol®)

- Beta blockers can slow the heart rate, and when taken in combination with other medications, such as the heart and blood pressure medications listed above, they may have an additive effect of *really* slowing the heart rate down or creating abnormal heart rhythms.

- The use of clonidine (Catapres) in combination with beta blockers has the potential to elevate blood pressure to unhealthy levels. If you are taking any of the above heart medications, monitor your heart rate and blood pressure closely.

- Cyclosporine (Neoral) and the fibrate medications listed above may increase the half-life of many beta blockers, increasing the risk of experiencing side effects.

- Anticonvulsants like phenobarbital (Luminal) can decrease the half-life of many beta blockers, rendering them less effective.

Diuretics

There are different classes of diuretics, also called "water pills," that differ depending on where they work in the kidney. Some diuretics are used primarily for the treatment of high blood pressure. Others are better at helping to treat swelling or edema. Yet others can positive effects on both and really help to protect the heart and even improve its function. Often people are prescribed more than one type of diuretic. As noted in the beginning of the chapter, they can increase the risk of developing dehydration and kidney and electrolyte issues, especially in the elderly population.

1 Which (if any) of the following diuretics are you currently taking?

☐ Hydrochlorothiazide (HCTZ)

☐ Chlorthalidone (Hygroton)

☐ Furosemide (Lasix)

☐ Bumetanide (Bumex®)

☐ Torsemide (Demadex)

☐ Spironolactone (Aldactone)

☐ Eplerenone (Inspra)

☐ Other: _____

2 Why have you been prescribed this medication?

☐ Hypertension

☐ CHF

☐ Heart disease

☐ Edema

☐ Problems with fluid overload

☐ Very low potassium level (hypokalemia)

☐ Very high potassium level (hyperkalemia)

☐ Other: _____

- Hydrochlorothiazide (HCTZ) and chlorthalidone (Hygroton) are both classified as the "thiazide type of diuretics" and they are used for the treatment of high blood pressure. If you have persistent problems with high potassium levels, they also can be prescribed for this purpose. They are usually taken once a day.

- Furosemide (Lasix), bumetanide (Bumex), and torsemide (Demadex) are examples of "loop diuretics." They are commonly prescribed for the treatment of edema and CHF. While they do have blood pressure–lowering effects, they are not believed to be as effective as the thiazide type of diuretics.

- Spironolactone (Aldactone) and eplerenone (Inspra) are "potassium-sparing diuretics." These medications have excellent blood pressure–lowering properties and are very heart protective. Many studies demonstrate the benefit of these medications in the treatment of CHF. Because they are potassium-sparing, they can raise potassium levels. For example, it is not uncommon to prescribe the loop diuretic furosemide (Lasix) and the potassium-sparing spironolactone together for the treatment of acute CHF, as furosemide's potassium-lowering and spironolactone's potassium-raising properties often balance each other out.

3 Have you experienced any of the following symptoms while taking this medication?

☐ Dry mouth

☐ Dizziness or lightheadedness

☐ Fatigue

☐ Generalized weakness

☐ Muscle weakness

☐ Breast or nipple tenderness

☐ Other: _____

- Diuretics can cause dehydration, which in turn can cause you to feel weak and tired. It is important to weigh yourself on a daily basis. Talk with your physician about weight guidelines. For example, if your weight drops below a set level, then perhaps you should discontinue the diuretic.

- Breast and/or nipple tenderness is a side effect associated with spironolactone (Aldactone). This can occur after starting the medication or increasing the dosage. Given the many potential benefits of this medication class, your physician may elect to prescribe eplerenone (Inspra), which does not have this side effect, if the tenderness is interfering with your quality of life.

4 **Have you had recent blood work to measure any or all of the following?**

☐ Sodium level

☐ Potassium level

☐ Magnesium level

☐ Creatinine level

- Fatigue and muscle weakness can be associated with dehydration or low levels of certain key minerals including potassium, magnesium, and even sodium. These blood levels should be monitored if you are taking a diuretic.

- Health professionals will often order a blood test called a "basic metabolic panel" or "chem 7." This test looks at seven basic elements of your blood chemistry, including sodium level, potassium level, and kidney function (creatinine level). Magnesium is not part of this lab panel and needs to be ordered separately.

- Often, low potassium is seen with low magnesium levels. Monitoring and replacing these key nutrients are important, because low levels can affect heart function.

- If you have been diagnosed with kidney problems, this may affect your ability to take potassium-sparing diuretics.

5 **Are you taking any of the following medications that might interact with diuretics?**

☐ NSAIDs such as ibuprofen or naproxen (Aleve)

☐ ARBs

☐ ACE Inhibitors

- ACE inhibitors and ARBs can worsen kidney function and can raise potassium levels in some individuals—a risk that increases if you are taking diuretics.

- The combination of taking NSAIDs and the ACE inhibitors/ARBs, and/or diuretics has the potential to worsen kidney function markedly and lower potassium levels. *If you develop any nausea, vomiting, diarrhea, or acute illness, call your doctor immediately as some or all of these drugs may need to be discontinued.*

✳ ✳ ✳

MEDICATION SPOTLIGHT

Loop Diuretics and "Sulfa" Allergies

Many medications, especially "sulfa antibiotics" such as Bactrim, are sulfa-derived, meaning they are made from or closely related to sulfanilamide. Loop diuretics are also "sulfa-related" medications. Just because someone is sulfa-allergic, however, does not always mean her or she cannot take a loop diuretic. Many patients with a sulfa allergy have been taking furosemide (Lasix) or another loop diuretic for years.

In the case that you have a true sulfa allergy, and you are not able to take any of the loop diuretics mentioned in this chapter, then you have another loop diuretic option: ethacrynic acid (Edecrin®). This is an older medication that can sometimes be tough for pharmacies to get, but if you have a sulfa allergy and you need to be on a diuretic, talk to your doctor about this medication.

✳ ✳ ✳

Alpha Blockers

Alpha blockers help small blood vessels remain open. They also have an inhibitory effect on the "fight or flight" hormone norepinephrine (noradrenaline). Because alpha blockers have this "relaxation effect" on other muscles throughout the body, these medications can help improve urine flow in older men with benign prostatic hyperplasia (BPH).

1 Which (if any) of the alpha blockers are you currently taking?

☐ Doxazosin (Cardura®)

☐ Tamsulosin (Flomax®)

☐ Terazosin (Hytrin®)

☐ Prazosin (Minipress®)

☐ Other: _____

- Tamsulosin (Flomax) is only prescribed for the treatment of BPH, as it has only a minimal effect on blood pressure.

2 Why have you been prescribed this medication?

☐ Hypertension

☐ BPH

☐ Other: _____

3 What dose are you taking, at what frequency?

_____ mg _____ times a day

4 Have you experienced any of the following symptoms while taking this medication?

☐ Lightheadedness when standing up (orthostatic hypotension)

☐ Edema

☐ Dizziness

☐ Drowsiness

☐ Headache

☐ Flushing of the skin

☐ Other: _____

- Orthostatic hypotension is a very common side effect with this class of medications, although it can occur with any blood pressure medication. Have your blood pressure checked in the sitting and standing positions. If you stand up and there is a significant difference in your blood pressure reading from when you were sitting, then medication adjustments may be needed.

- It is important to get up slowly after starting an alpha blocker.

- This class of medications can cause edema, although it is not a common side effect.

5 Are you taking any of the following medications that might interact with alpha blockers?

☐ Sildenafil (Viagra®)

☐ Macrolide antibiotics including erythromycin and clarithromycin (Biaxin)

☐ Other blood pressure medications in this chapter

- Medications such as sildenafil (Viagra) and other potent vasodilators can cause very low blood pressure in combination with any of the medications in this class.

- Macrolide antibiotics can interfere with the metabolism of the alpha blockers, increasing their half-life and worsening the side effect of low blood pressure.

- Note that low blood pressure can be a significant side effect when alpha blockers are taken in combination with any blood pressure–lowering medication in this chapter.

Nitrates

Nitrates are potent vasodilators that have a useful role in the management and treatment of angina (chest pain). Angina results from an inadequate supply of oxygen-carrying blood to the heart muscle via the coronary arteries. These medicines work by dilating veins and arteries and reducing the workload of the heart. The overall effect is the relief of episodes of chest pain. These medications are also used for the treatment of acute and chronic CHF. They have a blood pressure–lowering effect as well.

Nitrates can be taken long-term or on an as-needed basis, such as during or just before anticipated exercise, and they are available in several dosages and formulations (oral, sublingual, transdermal, and injections).

1 Which (if any) of the following nitrates are you currently taking?

☐ Isosorbide mononitrate (Imdur)

☐ Isosorbide dinitrate (Isordil)

☐ Sublingual (administered under the tongue) glyceryl trinitrate (GTN) pills or lingual spray

☐ Transdermal (GTN) patches/ointments

☐ Other: _____

- Isosorbide mononitrate (Imdur) tablets are used for long-term treatment of chronic angina, and they are usually taken every day. (Do not stop taking them unless your doctor tells you to or you develop intolerance.)

- GTN pills or spray is short acting and thus can be used for symptom relief, but it is not used for long-term treatment of angina. This medication comes in various forms, including tablets, sprays, and patches.

- Sublingual nitrate tablets should be placed under the tongue and allowed to dissolve. They must be stored in their original containers, away from humidity and moisture, and should not be crushed.

- A transdermal GTN patch should be reapplied daily to a new skin site and taken off for approximately eight hours (usually overnight) to prevent nitrate tolerance.

2 Have you experienced any of the following symptoms while taking this medication?

☐ Headache

☐ Low blood pressure (hypotension)

☐ Lightheadedness

☐ Passing out (syncope)

☐ Weakness

☐ Other: _____

- Many side effects of these medications are related to a drop in blood pressure, so make sure to check your blood pressure routinely.

- Do NOT drink alcohol if you are taking this class of medication, as it may cause a severe decrease in blood pressure (hypotension) and fainting spells (syncope).

3 Are you taking any of the following medications that might interact with nitrates?

☐ Calcium channel blockers (CCBs)

☐ Medications for erectile dysfunction such as sildenafil (Viagra), vardenafil (Levitra®), or tadalafil (Cialis®)

☐ Riociguat (Adempas®)

- Calcium channel blockers may increase the risk of developing orthostatic hypotension.

- Sildenafil (Viagra), vardenafil (Levitra), tadalafil (Cialis), and riociguat (Adempas) increase the hypotensive effect by relaxing the blood vessels, so avoid use of these medications within twenty-four hours of taking a nitrate.

- Please speak to your doctor about all your medications before starting any of the drugs mentioned above. It is an absolute no-no to take sildenafil (Viagra) or any similar variations of this medication while taking nitrates.

* * *

CONDITION SPOTLIGHT

Nitrate Tolerance

Continuous nitrate treatment leads to a tolerance of the drug within twenty-four to forty-eight hours, at which time normal doses of nitrates are no longer effective. Tolerance is a problem with long-acting nitrates (oral and transdermal forms), which is why a nitrate-free interval is necessary. However, nitrate tolerance does not usually develop with sublingual forms (tablets that dissolve under the tongue) of the medication.

The best way to avoid tolerance is to use long-acting nitrates intermittently, scheduling eight- to twelve-hour nitrate-free breaks, frequently done during periods of sleep. Some people notice that angina worsens during this nitrate-free period, which is a phenomenon called "rebound angina." This can be treated by increasing the dose of other drugs.

* * *

Clonidine (Catapres)

This medication is classified as an "alpha 2 agonist" because it is "centrally acting"—meaning it acts on alpha receptors located in the brain—to reduce blood pressure. Because of the significant side-effect profile, however, we tend to use these medications only when other medications are not effective in the treatment of high blood pressure.

1 Which (if any) of the following forms of clonidine are you currently taking?

☐ Pill

☐ Clonidine (Catapres) patch

☐ Other: _____

2 What dose are you currently taking, at what frequency?

_____ mg _____ times a day.

- Clonidine (Catapres) pills are dosed 0.1–0.2 mg and commonly prescribed to be taken two to three times a day, since it is a shorter-acting medication.

- The patch comes in doses of 0.1–0.3 mg but needs to be changed weekly. *If you are taking this medication, it is vital that you replace the patch on the same day each week.* This is because the patch works by building up to a therapeutic level in the body. Replacing it the same time each week maintains this consistent level in the body to help fight high blood pressure.

3 Have you experienced any of the following symptoms while taking this medication?

☐ Fatigue

☐ Sleepiness

☐ Confusion

☐ Dizziness

☐ Constipation

☐ Dry mouth

☐ Slow heart rate

☐ Skin rash (with the transdermal patch)

☐ Other: _____

- Known side effects of this medication include fatigue and sleepiness—even confusion and dizziness. Doctors are often very hesitant to prescribe this medication to the elderly because these side effects can be magnified.

- *Like beta blockers, these medications cannot be stopped "cold turkey,"
  because there is a risk of rebound hypertension.* Please speak with your
  physician before stopping this medication, as the dosage needs to be
  decreased slowly over a period of a few weeks.

- Many physicians prefer the patch because it can provide a continuous,
  level blood pressure over a twenty-four-hour period. If you are using
  the patch, you should rotate where you place it on your skin each
  week, as a common side effect is a rash over the site. If the rash is
  severe, you may need to change to the oral form.

4 Has your doctor spoken with you about making the transition to the patch?

☐ Yes.

☐ No.

- If you are on pills and you are going to make a transition to the patch,
  remember that it takes up to two days to achieve a therapeutic blood
  level of the medication. That means that you may need to take oral
  clonidine (Catapres) for two days after the patch is applied to the skin.

5 Are you taking any of the following medications that might interact with clonidine (Catapres)?

☐ Beta blockers such as metoprolol (Lopressor)

☐ Tricyclic antidepressants such as amitriptyline (Elavil®)

☐ Benzodiazepines including lorazepam (Ativan®) and diazepam
(Valium®)

- The combination of beta blockers and clonidine (Catapres) can
  increase the risk of developing high blood pressure in some individuals. This combination of medications can also decrease your pulse.

- If you are taking any of the tricyclic antidepressants with clonidine
  (Catapres), the combination may cause orthostatic hypotension (e.g.,
  dizziness when you stand up).

- Clonidine (Catapres) can also increase sedation and lethargy, so you
  need to be careful if you are taking any of the benzodiazepines. See
  chapter 5 for further information on these medications.

Notes

Warfarin & Other Blood Thinners

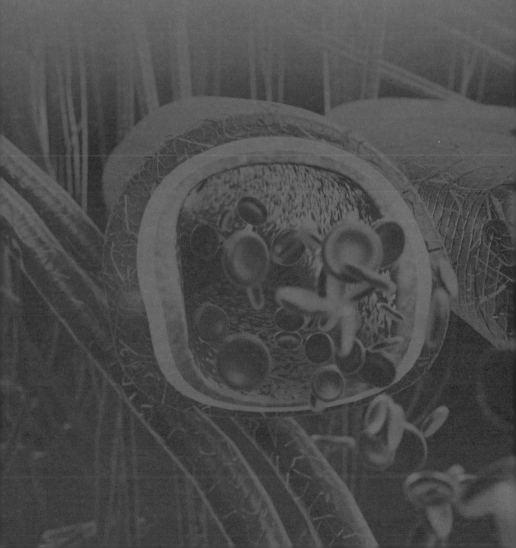

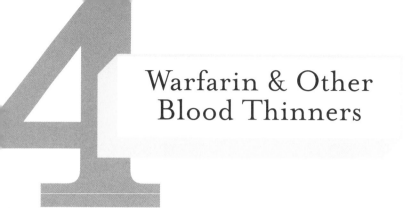

Warfarin & Other Blood Thinners

THIS CHAPTER CONCERNS THE USE OF MEDICATIONS THAT ARE used to thin the blood, also referred to as anticoagulation therapy. These agents will reduce the clotting ability of blood by increasing the time that blood takes to clot. Although they may not dissolve clots that are already formed, they are effective in preventing an existing blood clot (thrombus) from getting larger, as well as preventing new clots from forming.

Warfarin (Coumadin) has been around for a long time and is used to thin the blood for many conditions, including deep venous thrombosis (DVT), in which a blood clot forms in a leg vein; pulmonary embolism, which is a clot in the vessels of the lung; and atrial fibrillation, the most common abnormal heart rhythm. It is also used to prevent the formation of clots in those individuals with prosthetic valve replacements.

Warfarin requires constant monitoring through blood testing to be sure that the levels are not only therapeutic, but also safe. As you will read in this chapter, it does not take much for your warfarin levels to get out of whack, and many medications can interfere with its processing in the body. A change in your diet can affect warfarin levels, as can injury to your liver and/or acute intestinal illness. *The bottom line is that you need to be aware of just about everything you consume or experience while taking this medication.*

Novel oral anticoagulants (NOACs) are a newer class of blood thinners that are popular because they do not require the constant drug-level monitoring that warfarin does. That being said, they do have a significant side-effect profile and have not been studied in atypical patients or those in the extremes of body weight (warfarin has the advantage of being adjusted to a set level of anticoagulation and is preferred in atypical patients). Examples of the NOACs include dabigatran (Pradaxa®), rivaroxaban (Xarelto®), and apixaban (Eliquis).

Platelet inhibitors have been used for the treatment of acute heart attack and stroke. However, they also have a significant side-effect profile and can strongly interact with other medications. Many hospitals are conducting genetic testing for clopidogrel (Plavix), one of the most common antiplatelet agents utilized by physicians for the treatment of conditions including acute heart attack and stroke.

If you are admitted to the hospital for any acute medical condition, in all likelihood you will be given the blood thinner **heparin**. It is used to prevent the formation of blood clots while you are in the hospital, where you are not as mobile as you would be at home. It is also initially prescribed for the treatment of many of the acute problems that warfarin is used for, and it is even required to thin the blood in order to prepare a patient for warfarin therapy. As with the other anticoagulants, it is important to be aware of potential side effects of this medication.

It is no secret that the use of blood thinners puts patients at significant risk of bleeding. In addition to understanding the many potential interactions with blood thinners, we believe that understanding your own pharmacogenetic profile is also important. *If there is any chapter in this book that demonstrates the importance of personalizing the medication regimen to minimize risk and maximize patient safety, it is this one.* Dr. Khalighi and his team have done marvelous work on genotype profiling and certain blood thinners, including warfarin and clopidogrel (Plavix), and their results are shared in this chapter.

Warfarin (Coumadin)

Warfarin is one of the oldest blood thinners. It delays clot formation by inhibiting the production of vitamin K in the liver.

1 Why have you been prescribed warfarin?

☐ Atrial fibrillation

☐ Mechanical or tissue artificial heart valve

☐ DVT

☐ Pulmonary embolism

☐ A genetic clotting disorder

☐ Stroke

☐ Recent or previous heart attack

☐ Other: _____

- Understanding the reason why you are being prescribed warfarin helps to determine not only what its level needs to be in the blood but also how long you may need to take the medication. For example, if you have been diagnosed with DVT, the initial "duration of anticoagulation" might be three to six months. However, if there are some genetic factors that dramatically increase your risk of getting a clot, you might have to take warfarin for a longer period of time.

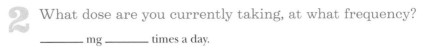

What dose are you currently taking, at what frequency?

_____ mg _____ times a day.

• Warfarin is often taken once daily. In terms of dosing, patients are conventionally started on a dose of 5 mg, and blood testing occurs daily with the goal of getting the international normalized ration (INR) to a certain level in three to four days. The long-term dose depends on how the patient processes warfarin in his or her body. Some people only require a daily dose of 1 mg while others might require a dose as high as 10 mg daily.

THE PERSONALIZED APPROACH

The Pharmacogenetics of Warfarin

Given the large variability in how people respond to different dosages of warfarin, it is often a challenge in clinical practice to find an appropriate dose for a patient, and frequent dose adjustments are often required. Fortunately, genetic testing is now available for personalized dosing, which decreases the risk of developing side effects. Warfarin works by suppressing an enzyme called VKORC1, which is deactivated by another enzyme called cytochrome CYP2C9. Recent advances in science have suggested that genetic variations of these two enzymes have a major effect on warfarin dosing.

Dr. Khalighi and his team have studied the DNA sequences of these enzymes in more than four hundred patients in his clinic. After analyzing individual genotype-specific warfarin dosing, they found that looking at individual genetic variations (polymorphisms) of the CYP2C9 and VKORC1 enzymes helped to improve the initial estimate of an appropriate warfarin dose, while also helping to identify "high risk" patients who need closer monitoring.

Before initiating warfarin therapy, your doctor may choose to analyze your CYP2C9 and VKORC1 enzyme activities to determine the appropriate warfarin dosage for you. Despite the promise of pharmacogenomics testing in warfarin dosing, its use in clinical practice is not universal, however.

3 The effectiveness of warfarin is most commonly measured by the prothrombin time (PT), how long it takes someone's blood to clot, which is then used to calculate the international normalized ratio (INR). How often do you have this test done?

- ☐ Once a week

- ☐ Once every two weeks

- ☐ Once a month

- ☐ Other: _____

- Since each person's liver metabolism and response to warfarin therapy is different, it is important to check INR more frequently when warfarin is first started or if there is a change in diet or certain medications.

- If your insurance approves it, you can get an INR tester/meter and do your own INR measurement in the comfort of your home. This sure beats going to the lab and getting blood drawn every time you need to have your warfarin level checked. If you don't have a tester/meter already, and you are on warfarin, call your doctor and/or your insurance company to see if you can get it.

* * *

MEDICATION SPOTLIGHT

Monitoring Your INR Value

Warfarin dosage is adjusted depending on your international normalized ratio (INR) value, which measures how long it takes for the blood to clot. For example, if your INR is 2, the blood is taking twice as long as normal to clot. The blood thinners are often prescribed when a patient's INR is between 2 and 3. If the INR is less than 2, the warfarin dose is increased; if it is more than 3, it is decreased. If you have a mechanical valve, however, your INR may be purposefully kept at 2.5–3.5.

* * *

4 Have you experienced any of the following symptoms while taking warfarin?

- ☐ Blood in your urine
- ☐ Bloody stools
- ☐ Easy bruising
- ☐ Bleeding when shaving
- ☐ Bleeding when brushing your teeth
- ☐ Coughing up blood
- ☐ Blood coming from your nose
- ☐ Other: _____

- *If you note any of the above bleeding events, you need to call your doctor right away and have your INR level checked.* If your INR is in the therapeutic range, you need to find out why you are bleeding.

- Blood in the urine suggests that there is an underlying issue in the genitourinary (GU) tract, meaning the kidneys, ureters, and/or bladder, while bloody stools indicate a problem with the gastrointestinal (GI) tract—that is, the intestine and colon. Your doctor may recommend further testing, including consultation with a gastroenterologist and/or a urologist.

- If you experience a bleeding event, your physician will have to assess bleeding risk compared to clotting risk. Your doctor may or may not be able to stop your warfarin based on this comparison. For example, if you have a heart valve replacement that is metallic, your doctor will not be able to stop your warfarin, as that can cause clots to form around the heart valve.

5 Do you have liver disease?

- ☐ Yes.
- ☐ No.
- ☐ I don't know.

- Warfarin interferes with vitamin K metabolism, which can cause elevations in the INR and increase the risk of bleeding. If you have advanced liver disease, your liver has problems making vitamin K in the first place.

Liver Disease

Major risk factors for liver disease in industrialized countries include obesity and diabetes, which increase the risk of developing a fatty liver and cirrhosis. Fatty liver is actually the leading cause of cirrhosis in industrialized countries, having replaced chronic alcohol use, which is now the second leading cause. Chronic use of acetaminophen may also have damaging effects to the liver, since it depletes an antioxidant called glutathione that is essential to the detoxification reaction in the body. See chapter 8 for more information on acetaminophen.

* * *

6 Do you eat roughly the same amount of green leafy vegetables or foods high in vitamin K every day?

☐ Yes.

☐ No.

- Certain foods with lots of vitamin K—such as spinach, kale, broccoli, mustard greens, collard greens, onions, brussels sprouts, and scallions— can reduce INR levels and affect warfarin metabolism.

- Eating a similar amount of vegetables and other foods that are high in vitamin K on a daily basis is essential if you are taking warfarin. *If you change your diet, please call your doctor, as your dosing may require adjustment, which will result in more frequent monitoring of your warfarin blood levels.*

- *Use of alcohol may affect the metabolism of warfarin and increase INR.*

7 Are you taking any of the following medications that might interact with warfarin?

☐ Aspirin

☐ NSAIDs such as ibuprofen or naproxen (Aleve)

☐ Other blood thinners mentioned in this chapter

☐ Amiodarone (Cordarone)

☐ Cimetidine (Tagamet®)

- [ ] Antibiotics such as levofloxacin (Levaquin®), ciprofloxacin (Cipro®), metronidazole (Flagyl®), erythromycin, sulfamethoxazole/trimethoprim (Bactrim), or fluconazole (Diflucan®)

- [ ] Prednisone (Deltasone®)

- [ ] Digoxin (Lanoxin)

- [ ] Mifepristone (Korlym®)

- [ ] Carbamazepine (Tegretol)

- Taking any combinations of blood thinners and/or aspirin or NSAIDs certainly increases the risk of bleeding.

- If you are taking any of the above drugs, check with your health-care professional, because you may be at a risk for increased bleeding or an abnormally high INR.

- Antibiotics can affect warfarin levels in a couple of ways: they can affect the intestinal processing of vitamin K, and they can also affect the liver processing of vitamin K. Your warfarin levels may need to be followed closely and your warfarin dosing decreased while you are on the antibiotic.

- If you are on warfarin and a new medication is being prescribed by any of your doctors, please talk with your pharmacist to see if there are any potential drug-drug interactions of which you need to be aware. While some medications may increase your INR, some—including broad-spectrum antibiotics and the anticonvulsant carbamazepine (Tegretol)—may decrease your INR.

Novel Oral Anticoagulants (NOACs)

The appeal of the medications in this increasingly popular class of blood thinners is that they don't require routine blood monitoring as warfarin does, yet they are prescribed for many of the same reasons that warfarin is.

1 Which (if any) of the following NOACs are you currently taking?

- [ ] Dabigatran (Pradaxa)

- [ ] Apixaban (Eliquis)

- [ ] Rivaroxaban (Xarelto)

- [ ] Edoxaban (Savaysa®)

☐ Other: _____

- The above anticoagulants all work differently and are metabolized differently. *You should not be taking more than one of these at the same time, as this will increase your risk of bleeding.*

2 Why have you been prescribed this medication?

☐ Preventing clot formation after knee/hip surgery (postoperative thromboprophylaxis)

☐ Prevent stroke due to atrial fibrillation or atrial flutter

☐ DVT

☐ Possible pulmonary embolism (PE)

☐ Genetic predisposition to clot formation

☐ Other: _____

- The NOACS are not intended for use by patients with prosthetic heart valves.

3 What dose are you currently taking, at what frequency?

_____ mg _____ times a day.

- All four NOACs listed are to be taken twice daily.

4 Do you have kidney disease?

☐ Yes

☐ No

- If your doctor wants to prescribe you a NOAC, he or she should order blood work that assesses your creatinine level, complete blood count (CBC), and liver function.

- The dosage of these medications may vary depending on the presence or absence of kidney disease.

- Apixaban (Eliquis) is preferred in patients with renal impairment, whereas rivaroxaban (Xarelto) is not recommended if there is any renal impairment. Dabigatran (Pradaxa) requires a dosage decrease if there is renal impairment.

5 Have you experienced any of the following symptoms while taking this medication?

☐ Bloody stools

☐ Blood in the urine

☐ Coughing up blood

☐ Easy bruising

☐ Nosebleed

☐ Bleeding when shaving

☐ Bleeding when brushing your teeth

☐ Other: _____

- *Call your doctor or get medical help right away if you have any of these signs or symptoms of bleeding:* unexpected bleeding or bleeding that lasts a long time, such as unusual bleeding from the gums, nosebleeds that happen often, or menstrual or vaginal bleeding that is heavier than normal; severe bleeding that you cannot control; red, pink, or brown urine; red or black stools that resemble tar; coughing up or vomiting blood or vomit that resembles coffee grounds; unexpected swelling or joint pain; headaches, dizziness, and/or weakness.

6 Are you taking any of the following medications that could potentially interact with NOACs and increase risk of bleeding?

☐ Aspirin

☐ Antiplatelet agents such as clopidogrel (Plavix), ticagrelor (Brilinta), or prasugrel (Effient®)

☐ NSAIDs such ibuprofen or naproxen (Aleve)

☐ Other blood thinners

- The use of anticoagulants while taking any of the above drugs can increase bleeding risk. Again, it is very important to speak with your physician concerning the use of more than one blood thinner.

Blood Thinner Antidotes

As opposed to warfarin, which may take three to five days to achieve a therapeutic level, all the new oral anticoagulants can achieve a therapeutic effect within a couple of hours after consumption. Currently, warfarin can be reversed with vitamin K, and dabigatran (Pradaxa) can be reversed with idarucizumab (Praxbind®). Andexanet alfa will likely be approved soon based on clinical trials showing it can reverse the effects of both rivaroxaban (Xarelto) and apixaban (Eliquis).

* * *

Platelet Inhibitors

These medications are important for the treatment of acute heart attack and acute stroke. While they are effective in preventing platelets from blocking an artery, they also have bleeding-related side effects and medication interactions of which you need to be aware.

1 Which (if any) of the following platelet inhibitors are you currently taking?

☐ Clopidogrel (Plavix)

☐ Prasugrel (Effient)

☐ Ticagrelor (Brilinta)

☐ Other: _____

2 Why have you been prescribed this medication?

☐ Heart attack (myocardial infarction)

☐ Acute coronary syndrome (unstable angina, severe heart artery narrowing/blockage)

☐ Stroke

☐ Peripheral vascular disease (PVD)

☐ Other: _____

3 What dose are you currently taking, at what frequency?

_____ mg _____ times a day.

The Pharmacogenetics of Clopidogrel

Clopidogrol (Plavix) is processed by the isoenzyme CYP2C19. The gene for this enzyme carries significant individual variations, which in turn results in varied efficacy among patients.

Dr. Khalighi and his team performed a study wherein the DNA sequences of the CYP2C19 genes of more than three hundred patients were studied. They found that up to 18.8 percent of patients had a genotype that results in higher-than-normal CYP2C19 enzymatic activities, and 19.8 percent of patients had lower-than-normal CYP2C19 enzymatic activities, both of which require either a change in dose or an alternative medication to achieve the full therapeutic effect of clopidegrol.

Please note that some hospitals may order this genetic test to determine how your liver processes this medication before prescribing either this medication or another platelet inhibitor.

4 Have you experienced any of the following symptoms while taking this medication?

☐ Unusual bleeding

☐ Easy bruising

☐ Pinpoint reddish spots on the skin (petechiae)

☐ Dark or bloody urine

☐ Other: _____

5 Are you taking any of the following medications that might interact with platelet inhibitors?

☐ Proton pump inhibitors (PPIs)

☐ Other blood thinners

☐ NSAIDs such as ibuprofen or naproxen (Aleve)

☐ Aspirin

☐ Antidepressants such as citalopram (Celexa®), duloxetine (Cymbalta®), fluoxetine (Prozac®), paroxetine (Paxil®), and many others

☐ Morphine

- Proton pump inhibitors (PPIs) may decrease the effectiveness of clopidogrel (Plavix). Because PPIs are among the most commonly prescribed medications by physicians for reflux and other stomach-related conditions, it is important to be aware of this interaction.

- If you are taking other blood thinners, it certainly can increase bleeding risk.

- Please minimize the use of NSAIDs if you are taking platelet inhibitors or any other medications in this chapter, as the risk of bleeding, especially from the gastrointestinal tract, is significantly increased.

- The use of aspirin can increase bleeding risk as well, so aspirin will only be given to those taking blood platelet inhibitors in acute emergency situations, such as a major heart attack.

- The use of many antidepressants—including citalopram (Celexa), duloxetine (Cymbalta), escitalopram (Lexapro®), fluoxetine (Prozac), fluvoxamine (Luvox®), paroxetine (Paxil), sertraline (Zoloft®), trazodone (Oleptro®), venlafaxine (Effexor®), and others—with blood platelet inhibitors may impact the effectiveness of the inhibitors.

- The use of morphine may decrease the efficacy of blood platelet inhibitors, especially when it is given intravenously in a hospital.

Heparin

If you need to be hospitalized for any reason, one of the significant concerns of physicians is that you do not develop a clot while in the hospital. In fact, clot prevention is one of the "core measures" that every hospital abides by when taking care of patients. The other name for clot prevention is "DVT prophylaxis." Heparin or a derivative of heparin is administered under the skin (i.e., subcutaneously) by nurses for this reason.

1 Which (if any) of the following anticoagulants were you given for DVT prophylaxis?

☐ Heparin

☐ Enoxaparin (Lovenox®)

☐ Fondaparinux (Arixtra®)

☐ Other: _____

- Heparin is an injection that needs to be given three times a day in the hospital.

- Enoxaparin (Lovenox) is known as an "unfractionated heparin." It is given under the skin and requires only a once daily dosing.

- Fondaparinux (Arixtra) is an injection given under the skin and requires once daily dosing. It is often prescribed to prevent blood clots in individuals who are undergoing joint replacement surgery.

- Your renal function will determine whether you receive Lovenox or Arixtra versus heparin. Lovenox and Arixtra are not prescribed if there is advanced kidney disease present, which can increase bleeding risk. Heparin, on the other hand, can be given safely if there is kidney disease present.

2 Have you been hospitalized for an acute DVT or an acute pulmonary embolism?

☐ Yes.

☐ No.

- Just as an acute DVT is a clot that occurs in the deep leg veins, an acute pulmonary embolism (PE) is a clot in the pulmonary artery or one of its branches in a lung. The goal of anticoagulation is to prevent further blood clots from forming as well as preventing the current clot from getting bigger.

- If you have a DVT and/or PE, your physician will discuss various options in what type of anticoagulation you may receive. One option is placement of a continuous intravenous heparin infusion. A blood test called a PTT is given every six hours to ensure that the blood is thin enough but not too thin. After being on heparin for twenty-four to forty-eight hours, a transition to warfarin may occur.

Notes

Notes

Medications
& the
Psyche

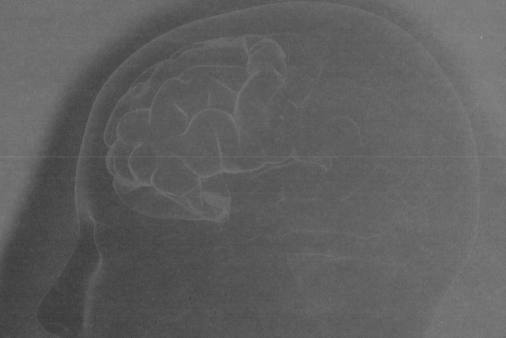

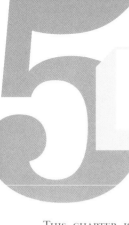

Medications &
the Psyche

This chapter is dedicated to discussing medications prescribed for brain-related illnesses and conditions. This includes prescriptions for everything from seizures to depression, as well as medications that may be used "off-label" for other conditions. One of the most common examples of off-label use is the prescribing of antiseizure medications for the treatment of neuropathic pain. (See chapter 8 for further information concerning pain-related medications.)

The medication types featured in this chapter include **antiseizure medications** (also known as anticonvulsants and anti-epileptics), such as the classic phenytoin (Dilantin®) and phenobarbital (Luminal), as well as newer medications like levetiracetam (Keppra®) and lamotrigine (Lamictal®). Many of the medications in this class can have significant side effects and influence the processing of other medications (and each other). Antiseizure medications also affect vitamin D metabolism and, thus, bone health.

Antipsychotics are effective but also associated with a list of side effects, including increased risk of diabetes and high cholesterol and triglyceride levels. We will focus on the more common antipsychotics, including haloperidol (Haldol®), olanzapine (Zyprexa®), and clozapine (Clozaril®).

In 2013, antidepressants were the most commonly prescribed medication in the United States. There are several classes of antidepressants used in the treatment of depression. These classes include the **selective serotonin reuptake inhibitors (SSRIs)** and **tricyclics**. Commonly prescribed SSRIs include sertraline (Zoloft), citalopram (Celexa), paroxetine (Paxil), and fluoxetine (Prozac). Common tricyclic antidepressants include amitriptyline (Elavil) and nortriptyline (Pamelor®).

Medications used for the treatment of anxiety and sleep disorders include a class of medications called **benzodiazepines**, which are also prescribed for the treatment of acute seizures. Popular "benzos" include lorazepam (Ativan) and alprazolam (Xanax®). Other medications used specifically to combat insomnia include **sleep aids** like zolpidem (Ambien®).

Note that many of the medications in this chapter can be used for more than one condition. For example, the benzodiazepines can be used for the treatment of anxiety as well as seizures, and antidepressants can be used for the treatment of chronic pain and anxiety. Also, while many primary care physicians are comfortable prescribing some antidepressants, many of the medications in this chapter are usually prescribed by specialists. For example, neurologists more commonly prescribe antiseizure medications, and psychiatrists are more comfortable and familiar with prescribing antipsychotic, antianxiety, and other medication classes mentioned in this chapter.

WARNING

Many of the medications discussed in this chapter cannot be abruptly stopped. If a medication needs to be discontinued, its dosage needs to be decreased slowly over a period of time. If another medication is to be started in its place, your doctor will likely start the new medication at a low dose and slowly increase it while simultaneously decreasing the old medication. This is especially true for antiseizure and antidepressant medications.

Also, please refrain from drinking alcohol while taking medications listed in this chapter—particularly the benzodiazepines and sedatives like zolpidem (Ambien) and phenobarbital (Luminal), as the combination can be lethal. Alcohol can also lower your seizure threshold, i.e., it can increase your risk of having a seizure if you have an underlying seizure disorder. If you are on an antidepressant medication, realize that alcohol is a "brain depressant" and can thus counter the effects of the antidepressant.

Antiseizure Medications

Below are the most commonly prescribed medications for the treatment of seizures and seizure disorders. In many instances, more than one medication may be prescribed to help manage this condition effectively.

1 Which (if any) of the following anticonvulsants are you currently taking? (Check all that apply.)

- ☐ Phenytoin (Dilantin)
- ☐ Phenobarbital (Luminal)
- ☐ Lamotrigine (Lamictal)
- ☐ Valproic acid (Depakote®)
- ☐ Levetiracetam (Keppra)
- ☐ Carbamazepine (Tegretol)

☐ Oxcarbazepine (Trileptal®)

☐ Gabapentin (Neurontin®)

☐ Other: _____

- Lamotrigine (Lamictal) and valproic acid (Depakote) are also prescribed for the treatment of manic-depressive disorder.

- Carbamazepine (Tegretol) and oxcarbazepine (Trileptal) have also been prescribed for the treatment of trigeminal neuralgia and neuropathy.

2 What dose are you currently taking, at what frequency?

_____ mg _____ times a day.

· ·

THE PERSONALIZED APPROACH
Anticonvulsives for Neuropathy

Nowhere is personalized dosing more prevalent than in the dosing of anti-seizure medications. For example, some of these medications have been prescribed for the treatment of pain, and some people may require high dosages for effective pain relief. At higher doses, however, side effects are expected. For example, high doses of carbamazepine (Tegretol) have been used for the treatment of painful neuropathy, and it is expected that low sodium levels may occur in some individuals.

For many people, it may take a long time for pain to be effectively controlled by anticonvulsives. *We cannot emphasize enough the importance of shared decision-making when it comes to the prescription and dosing of medications.*

· ·

3 Have you experienced any of the following symptoms while taking this medication(s)?

☐ Dizziness

☐ Jerking of the arms and/or legs

☐ Nausea

☐ Vomiting

☐ Lethargy

☐ Confusion

☐ Increased sleep

☐ Other: _____

- Phenytoin (Dilantin) is commonly given in the hospital for the treatment of acute seizures, but it has many possible side effects including dizziness, lightheadedness, and gingival hyperplasia (big gums).

- *Signs and symptoms of phenytoin (Dilantin) toxicity include lethargy, hypotension (low blood pressure), jerking movements of the hands, difficulty walking, and slurring of speech that mimics an acute stroke. Significant nausea and vomiting, and even coma, have been reported.*

- Potential side effects of phenobarbital (Luminal) include lethargy, problems with memory, and changes in behavior.

- Potential side effects of valproic acid (Depakote) include increased liver enzymes and pancreatitis.

- A significant side effect of valproic acid (Depakote), carbamazepine (Tegretol), and oxcarbazepine (Trileptal) is hyponatremia (low sodium level). If you are taking one of these medications, your health-care provider will likely order routine blood tests to analyze your sodium level, especially if your dosage is being increased. Low sodium levels are not as common with valproic acid (Depakote), but the effect has been reported. *Extremely low sodium levels can cause confusion, lethargy, and a serious condition that can impair thinking and brain functioning.*

- The most common side effects of gabapentin (Neurontin) include dizziness, fatigue, weight gain, and swelling of the extremities, but sexual dysfunction has also been reported.

* * *

CONDITION SPOTLIGHT

Psycholeptic Toxicity

Many of the medications discussed in this chapter are *psycholeptics*—that is, they exude a calming effect on individuals. In addition to alcohol and opiates (whether illicit or prescribed), these substances consist of barbiturates (e.g., phenobarbital), antipsychotics, benzodiazepines, antihistamines, and sleep aids such as zolpidem (Ambien). Because such drugs depress the central nervous system, care must be taken that they are not taken in excess or in combination with one another, as toxic doses can be fatal. *If you have taken more than the prescribed dose of your psycholeptic and/or in combination with other psycholeptics, including alcohol or opiates, and you experience severe lethargy, difficulty walking, impaired speech, and/or double vision, please get immediate help.*

* * *

4 Does your medication(s) require regular monitoring of drug levels in the blood?

☐ Yes.

☐ No.

☐ I don't know.

- Phenytoin (Dilantin), phenobarbital (Luminal), carbamazepine (Tegretol), and valproic acid (Depakote) blood levels are routinely monitored to ensure that you are taking a safe dose.

- Gabapentin (Neurontin) and levetiracetam (Keppra) levels can be monitored, but this is not common practice, especially at low doses.

- Phenytoin (Dilantin) toxicity can occur with a blood concentration above 20 μg/ml.

- Phenytoin (Dilantin) and phenobarbital (Luminal) are "enzyme inducers," meaning that they increase the liver processing and decrease the levels of other medications in the body, including other seizure medications. They can even decrease the levels of each other.

5 Do you have abnormal kidney or liver function?

☐ Yes.

☐ No.

☐ I don't know.

- Levetiracetam (Keppra) and gabapentin (Neurontin) need to be dosed according to your kidney function level; if your kidney function is not normal, your dosage will be decreased.

- Many antiseizure medications, with the exception of gabapentin (Neurontin), are processed in the liver. If your liver function is compromised, many of the above medications may not be prescribed, need to be discontinued, or have their dosages drastically reduced.

Vitamin D

Phenytoin (Dilantin) and phenobarbital (Luminal) can decrease the levels of vitamin D in the blood. Many people take medications like Dilantin for years, and thus have chronic low vitamin D levels, which affect bone health and are a risk factor for the development of osteoporosis. Low vitamin D levels have also been found in patients taking valproic acid (Depakote), oxcarbazepine (Trileptal), and carbamazepine (Tegretol). For the many people on multiple antiseizure medications, the effect of vitamin D deficiency is amplified. *Supplementation with vitamin D, and even bisphosphonates, is essential if you are taking antiseizure medications. This is especially important for children, whose bones are still growing.* See chapter 10 for information concerning vitamin D types and dosage.

* * *

6 Are you taking any of the following medications that might interact with antiseizure medications?

☐ Fluconazole (Diflucan)

☐ Cimetidine (Tagamet)

☐ Sulfamethoxazole/trimethoprim (Bactrim)

☐ Amiodarone (Cordarone)

☐ Warfarin

- The medications above, while not an exhaustive list, can interfere with the liver processing of other antiseizure medications.

- Fluconazole (Diflucan, an antifungal) and cimetidine (Tagamet, used for the treatment of heartburn and ulcers) are enzymatic inhibitors that can interfere with the metabolism of many antiseizure medications.

- Many of the antiseizure medications in this chapter can also affect the processing of warfarin. Phenytoin (Dilantin) and phenobarbital (Luminal), for example, can decrease the length of time warfarin is in the body.

- Amiodarone (Cordarone), commonly prescribed for the treatment of abnormal heart rhythms, can increase levels of certain medications, including phenytoin (Dilantin), in the body.

- Sulfamethoxazole/trimethoprim (Bactrim), like phenytoin (Dilantin) and warfarin, is processed in the liver by the CYP2C9 pathway, and as an inhibitor of this pathway, it can increase levels of these medications in the body.

7 Are either of the following part of your regular diet or supplement regimen?

☐ Grapefruit or grapefruit juice

☐ St John's wort

- Be aware that grapefruit can inhibit the processing of many medications by the liver, so its consumption should be limited.

- St John's wort has the effect of being an enzymatic inducer; that is, it can speed up the processing of many medications in the liver and decrease their blood levels more quickly. We recommend limiting the use of this supplement if you are on multiple medications, especially the ones discussed in this chapter.

Selective Serotonin Reuptake Inhibitors (SSRIs)

These are among the most popular medications prescribed for the treatment of depression—particularly major depressive disorder—but they can help alleviate anxiety as well. They are very effective, and many of the side effects are tolerable.

1 Which (if any) of the following SSRIs are you currently taking?

☐ Sertraline (Zoloft)

☐ Citalopram (Celexa)

☐ Escitalopram (Lexapro)

☐ Fluoxetine (Prozac)

☐ Paroxetine (Paxil)

☐ Fluvoxamine (Luvox)

☐ Other: _____

2 What dose are you currently taking, at what frequency?

_____ mg _____ times a day.

- The medications in this class are commonly taken once per day, beginning at a low dose that is increased slowly.

- The initial dose for sertraline (Zoloft) is 25 mg daily and doses can range up to 100 mg; paroxetine (Paxil) and citalopram (Celexa) are usually started at 10 mg daily.

3 Have you experienced any of the following symptoms while taking this medication?

☐ Increased sleep

☐ Insomnia

☐ Weight loss

☐ Weight gain

☐ Sexual dysfunction and/or loss of libido

☐ Thoughts of suicide

☐ Dizziness

☐ Nausea

☐ Lethargy

☐ Confusion

☐ Other: _____

- Changes in sleep and weight are common side effects of these medications. If any of the medications in this class cause you to sleep more, your doctor may suggest that you take these medications before going to sleep. If, on the other hand, your medication causes insomnia, your doctor may suggest taking your medication in the morning.

- Sexual side effects can occur in men and women. The range of side effects include loss of sexual interest and inability to achieve an orgasm. One study suggested that paroxetine (Paxil) may be associated with more severe sexual side effects compared to the other medications in this class.

- Paradoxically, a potential side effect of the SSRIs is suicidal ideation, though this is more commonly observed in adolescents and young adults. This risk may be increased by sunshine, believe it or not. A study from the *Journal of Affective Disorders* in October 2015 found that there was a clear association between the effects of the sun and increased risk of suicide in those taking SSRIs. *Again, because of the effects that these medications have on brain chemistry, they cannot be stopped abruptly, but if you are having any suicidal thoughts, you need to get help immediately.*

....

THE PERSONALIZED APPROACH

SSRIs and Genetic Testing

Genetic testing can show how well your liver is able to utilize its CYP2D6 and CYP2C19 pathways, which SSRIs may inhibit. If you are a slow metabolizer of this metabolic pathway, it means that medications using this pathway may hang around longer, which can increase the risk of developing side effects. The most potent inhibitors of the CYP2D6 pathway include paroxetine (Paxil) and fluoxetine (Prozac). Sertraline (Zoloft) seems to be in the middle, while citalopram (Celexa) and fluvoxamine (Luvox) have the least effect. This means you should stay away from paroxetine or fluoxetine in particular if you are found to be a poor metabolizer of the CYP2D6 pathway. You can see that between your own "liver phenotype" and the effects medications such as these have on your liver, a "double whammy" can occur, potentially increasing your experience of negative side effects.

....

4 Are you taking any of the following medications that might interact with SSRIs?

☐ Clopidogrel (Plavix)

☐ Tramadol (Ultram)

☐ Diphenhydramine (Benadryl®)

☐ Triptans such as sumatriptan (Imitrex®)

☐ Dextromethorphan-containing cough suppressants

☐ Tricyclic antidepressants

☐ Other reuptake inhibitors

☐ Other: _____

- As you may have read in chapter 4, clopidogrel (Plavix) requires the processing of the CYP2C19 pathway in order for the medication to be "activated." Certain SSRIs, such as fluvoxamine (Luvox), may delay this processing, meaning that it may take longer for Plavix to be effective as an antiplatelet agent in some people.

* * *

Serotonin Syndrome

Serotonin syndrome is a very dangerous and potentially fatal reaction characterized by increased heart rate, overactive reflexes or involuntary muscle twitching, and hyperthermia. This syndrome can be brought on by an interaction between medications that increase serotonin levels in the body. This encompasses the SSRIs in combination with a number of different medications, including: tricyclic antidepressants; tramadol (an opioid pain medication); the class of medications known as the triptans (for headaches); over-the-counter cold and cough medicines that contain dextromethorphan (including such brands as Robitussin®, NyQuil®, and TheraFlu®); diphenhydramine (Benadryl); and other psychoactive medications including valproic acid (Depakote). *If you are prescribed any medication that works through regulation of serotonin levels in the brain, you need to check with your doctor or pharmacist to see if other medications you are taking could potentially produce this serious interaction. If you experience any of the symptoms listed above, please contact your doctor immediately.* The bottom line is that when it comes to medications that can affect brain chemistry, you need to be extra vigilant to prevent or manage potential drug-drug interactions.

* * *

Other Reuptake Inhibitors

The medications in this group affect the serotonin and/or norepinephrine or dopamine receptors. They include some of the most recent drugs developed for the treatment of depression.

1 Which (if any) of the following reuptake inhibitors are you currently taking?

☐ Venlafaxine (Effexor)

☐ Mirtazapine (Remeron®)

☐ Bupropion (Wellbutrin®)

☐ Nefazodone (Serzone®)

☐ Trazodone (Oleptro)

☐ Other: _____

- Venlafaxine (Effexor) is a serotonin-norepinephrine reuptake inhibitor (SNRI). Bupropion (Wellbutrin) works by affecting the reuptake of norepinephrine and dopamine. Nefazodone (Serzone) (weakly) affects the uptake of all three neurotransmitters, dopamine, norepinephrine, and serotonin.

- Trazodone (Oleptro) has some effect on serotonin, but a weaker effect compared to the other medications described above.

2 What dose are you currently taking, at what frequency?

_____ mg _____ times a day.

3 Have you experienced any of the following symptoms while taking this medication?

☐ High blood pressure

☐ Suicidal thoughts

☐ Dizziness

☐ Nausea

☐ Lethargy

☐ Confusion

☐ Increased sleep

☐ Insomnia

☐ Weight loss

☐ Weight gain

☐ Sexual side effects

☐ Orthostatic hypotension

☐ Other: _____

- Venlafaxine (Effexor) can increase your blood pressure, so you should monitor it while taking this medication. One study commented that suicide might be a potential side effect of this medication.

- Bupropion (Wellbutrin) can lower seizure threshold in susceptible individuals; if you have a history of seizures, then this may not be the best drug for you.

- Trazodone (Oleptro) can cause dizziness when standing up, a side effect called "postural hypotension."

4 Are you taking any of the following medications that might interact with reuptake inhibitors?

☐ Any SSRIs

☐ Macrolide antibiotics such as erythromycin

☐ Statins such as simvastatin (Zocor) and atorvastatin (Lipitor)

- Note that trazodone (Oleptro) is processed in the liver by the CYP3A4 pathway, so be aware of other medications that can affect this pathway, including macrolide antibiotics such as erythromycin. The statins simvastatin (Zocor) and atorvastatin (Lipitor) are also processed by CYP3A4 and may interact with this medication.

- Venlafaxine (Effexor) is processed in the liver by CYP2C19 and CYP2D6, and in some individuals it may have an increased propensity to interact with other medications compared to other antidepressants.

- Some of these medications, including venlafaxine (Effexor), bupropion (Wellbutrin), and trazodone (Oleptro), can increase the risk of developing serotonin syndrome, especially if taken in conjunction with other serotonin-affecting medications. See page 83.

Tricyclic Antidepressants

These medications are still commonly used for the treatment of depression. They can have other uses as well, however, including the treatment of pain and neuropathy (please see chapter 8 for further discussion). Also, it is not uncommon for a physician to prescribe an SSRI along with a tricyclic for the treatment of depression.

1 Which (if any) of the following tricyclics are you currently taking?

☐ Nortriptyline (Pamelor)

☐ Amitriptyline (Elavil)

☐ Imipramine (Tofranil®)

☐ Desipramine (Norpramin®)

☐ Doxepin (Sinequan®)

☐ Other: _____

2 What dose are you currently taking, at what frequency?

_____ mg _____ times a day.

3 Have you experienced any of the following symptoms while taking this medication?

☐ Constipation

☐ Dry eyes

☐ Difficulty urinating

☐ Postural hypotension

☐ Confusion

☐ Lethargy

☐ Dizziness

☐ Abnormal heart rhythms such as slow heart rate and/or palpitations

☐ Other: _____

- This class of medications can have what is called "anticholinergic properties," inhibiting nerve impulses of the parasympathetic nervous system, especially at higher doses. This can cause constipation, dry eyes, and difficulty urinating (due to urinary retention). They are also known to cause confusion.

- Tricyclics can also cause postural hypotension in some people.

- If you have a history of heart issues, a baseline EKG should be considered to evaluate if these medications could put you at risk of developing a cardiac arrhythmia (abnormal rhythm of the heart).

4 Are you taking any of the following medications that might interact with tricyclics?

☐ Any SSRIs

☐ Tramadol (Ultram)

- Tricyclic antidepressants are all metabolized by the CYP2D6 pathway and have the potential to interact with one another. The combination of tricyclic antidepressants and SSRIs can increase the risk of developing side effects including cardiac arrhythmias. As described on page 83, the combination of tricyclic antidepressants or SSRIs with tramadol increases the risk of developing serotonin syndrome.

Antipsychotic Medications

These medications are commonly prescribed for the treatment of acute psychosis, characterized by severe agitation, hallucinations, loss of contact with reality, paranoia, and bizarre behavior. Note that psychoses can be a spontaneous response to stress or trauma or an aspect of chronic conditions such as bipolar disorder or schizophrenia.

1 Which (if any) of the following antipsychotics are you currently taking?

- ☐ Haloperidol (Haldol)
- ☐ Risperidone (RisperDAL®)
- ☐ Olanzapine (ZyPREXA)
- ☐ Clozapine (Clozaril)
- ☐ Ziprasidone (Geodon®)
- ☐ Other: _____

2 What dose are you currently taking. at what frequency?

_____ mg _____ times a day.

3 Have you experienced any of the following symptoms while taking this medication?

- ☐ Lip smacking
- ☐ Involuntary muscle jerking
- ☐ Weight gain
- ☐ Dizziness
- ☐ Sleepiness
- ☐ Confusion
- ☐ Other: _____

- Antipsychotics work by blocking the dopamine receptors in the brain. It is the blocking of these receptors that produces many of the involuntary movements listed above. These symptoms are thought to be less likely with many of the newer medications in this group, including olanzapine (ZyPREXA) and clozapine (Clozaril).

- These medications have the propensity to cause weight gain as a side effect. It is important to watch your caloric intake and try to exercise regularly, especially since they can increase your risk of developing high cholesterol and triglyceride levels. In addition, they can also increase your risk of developing type 2 diabetes.

- Ziprasidone (Geodon) may have less of an impact on weight compared to the other atypical antipsychotics.

4 Are you taking any of the following medications that may interact with antipsychotics?

- ☐ Tricyclic antidepressants

- ☐ SSRIs

- ☐ Tramadol (Ultram)

- ☐ Duloxetine (Cymbalta)

- Antipsychotic medications, including risperidone (RisperDAL) and haloperidol (Haldol), are processed by the CYP2D6 pathway. Medications like SSRIs may inhibit or slow down this pathway, which can increase the risk of developing side effects.

- The use of antipsychotics in conjunction with SSRIs can not only increase the risk of developing serotonin syndrome, but also increase the risk of a condition called "neuroleptic malignant syndrome." Symptoms include fever, high or low blood pressure, and severe muscle rigidity. *If you are experiencing any of these symptoms, you need to call 911 right away.*

Benzodiazepines

Some of these medications, prescribed primarily for the treatment of anxiety and panic attacks, also may be prescribed for the treatment of sleeplessness. Benzodiazepines, or "benzos," such as lorazepam (Ativan) and clonazepam (Klonopin®), are also prescribed for the treatment of acute seizures. While they can be effective, physicians are very much aware of the potential for serious side effects, especially in elderly patients. These can include lethargy, confusion, and fatigue. Benzos can also be addictive, so many health professionals prefer to prescribe them for short-term use (a few weeks to a couple of months) or to be taken only occasionally, "as needed." If you need to be on these medications for a longer duration, you will have to be closely monitored by your physician, who may recommend that you see a specialist.

1 Which (if any) of the following medications are you currently taking?

☐ Alprazolam (Xanax)

☐ Lorazepam (Ativan)

☐ Temazepam (Restoril®)

☐ Clonazepam (Klonopin)

☐ Other: _____

2 What dose are you currently taking, at what frequency?

_____ mg _____ times a day.

- Alprazolam (Xanax) can be taken multiple times a day, with the lowest dose starting at 0.25 mg.

- Lorazepam (Ativan) can also be taken multiple times a day, the lowest dose being 0.5 mg.

3 Do you have liver disease?

☐ Yes.

☐ No.

☐ I don't know.

- Because many of these medications are processed by the liver, their half-life can be dramatically increased in the setting of advanced liver disease. If you absolutely need this medication, then you may need to start at a low dose or low frequency of dosage.

- Since they are not metabolized by CYP3A4, lorazepam (Ativan) and temazapam (Restoril) may be safer options for patients with liver disease.

4 Have you experienced any of the following symptoms while taking this medication?

☐ Confusion

☐ Lethargy

- [ ] Fatigue
- [ ] Agitation
- [ ] Hallucinations
- [ ] Insomnia
- [ ] Other: _____

- Benzodiazepines as a class can cause sedation, confusion, and lethargy. Because they are depressants of the central nervous system (CNS), you must speak with your doctor if you are operating heavy machinery or driving. You may have to take these medications at specific times during the day.

- These medications can also cause the symptoms of agitation, restlessness, and difficulty sleeping. This is called "paradoxical excitation," and it is more common in elderly patients. If any medications from this class are needed, patients (particularly the elderly) should take only the lowest dose possible.

5 Are you taking any of the following medications that might interact with benzodiazepines?

- [ ] Strong pain medications including tramadol (Ultram) and opiates such as oxycodone (OxyContin)

- [ ] Antiseizure medications

- [ ] Zolpidem (Ambien)

- [ ] Sedating antihistamines such as diphenhydramine (Benadryl) and doxylamine (Unisom®).

- The elderly should be particularly mindful of these interactions, which increase risk for falls.

- The combination of benzodiazepines with strong pain medications, such as opiates and tramadol (Ultram), can increase the risk of lethargy, confusion, and depression of the respiratory drive—with potentially fatal effects. Sedating antihistamines, sleep aids, and anticonvulsants increase this risk.

CONDITION SPOTLIGHT

Benzodiazepine Overdose

As mentioned, combining benzodiazepines with certain other drugs that have sedative properties can lead to fatal respiratory depression, but taking too high of a dose of these medications can have the same effect. Luckily, flumazenil (Romazicon®) has been developed as an antidote for acute benzodiazepine overdose. That said, if you have been on benzodiazepines for a long time or are prone to seizures, physicians may be hesitant about using this antidote unless absolutely necessary as blocking the receptor sites in the brain for a chronic benzodiazepine user can result in withdrawal symptoms such as seizures and potentially fatal cardiac effects.

* * *

Sleep Aids

While some benzodiazepines are used to combat insomnia, many over-the-counter antihistamines are also effective. More targeted sleep aids, such as zolpidem (Ambien), are also available.

1 Are you taking any of the following sleep aids?

☐ Zolpidem (Ambien)

☐ Diphenhydramine (Benadryl)

☐ Other: _____

2 What dose are you currently taking, at what frequency?

_____ mg _____ times a day.

- Zolpidem (Ambien) comes in a 5 and 10 mg dosing. If you are a male, you can be take up to 10 mg a day. If you are a female, you should not dose any higher than 5 mg. This is across the board, regardless of underlying personalized pharmacokinetics. Certain studies have demonstrated that females metabolize this medication slower than men, and thus, a reduced dosage is necessary to minimize side effects.

3 Have you experienced any of the following symptoms while taking this medication?

- ☐ Confusion
- ☐ Lethargy
- ☐ Fatigue
- ☐ Agitation
- ☐ Hallucinations
- ☐ Insomnia
- ☐ Orthostatic hypotension
- ☐ Urinary retention
- ☐ Other: _____

- Zolpidem (Ambien) has the same side-effect profile as benzodiazepines, including the risk of paradoxical excitation in elderly patients.

- Diphenhydramine (Benadryl) may cause dizziness when standing up (orthostatic hypotension) and urinary retention.

4 Are you taking any of the following medications that might interact with sleep aids?

- ☐ Strong pain medications including tramadol (Ultram) and opiates such as oxycodone (OxyContin)
- ☐ Antiseizure medications
- ☐ Benzodiazepines

- If you are taking a benzodiazepine already, taking sleep aids such as diphenhydramine (Benadryl) or zolpidem (Ambien) can be dangerous, as they very much increase the risk of developing lethargy and confusion, as well as depressing the respiratory drive, especially in elderly patients.

- Sedating pain medications should be avoided or limited for the same reasons that benzodiazepine–sleep aid and anticonvulsant–sleep aid combinations should.

SUPPLEMENT SPOTLIGHT

Melatonin

Melatonin is a popular over-the-counter supplement used to help people get to sleep. This supplement should be started at a low dose (e.g., 1 mg), especially if you are on medications discussed in this chapter. *Be sure to talk with your physician first if you are going to start any over-the-counter supplement in combination with any of the psychoactive medications.* Also, be aware that medications such as SSRIs can delay the processing of melatonin, leading to side effects like lightheadedness, irritable mood, and mild stomach upset. It may also cause increased lethargy the following day.

* * *

Notes

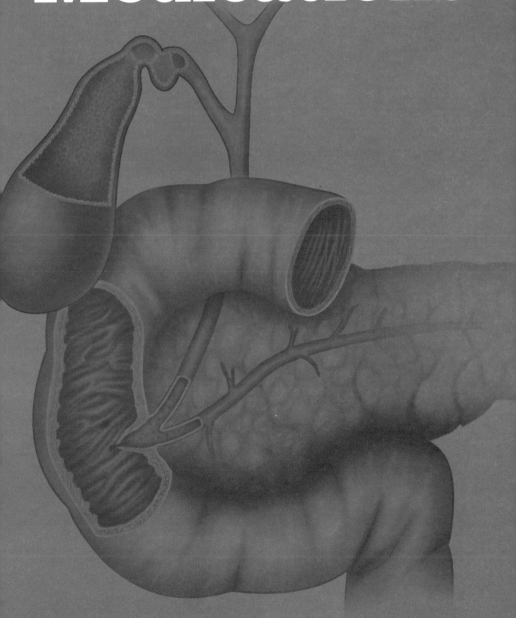

Diabetes
Medications

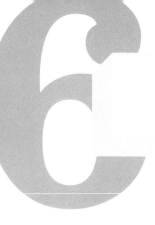

Diabetes Medications

IN ORDER FOR THE BODY TO WORK PROPERLY, it needs energy. Glucose is a primary fuel for the body and the only fuel for the brain. Insulin, a substance produced by the pancreas, is like a key that allows glucose to enter the body's cells. When glucose is not able to enter cells, either because of insulin resistance or a total absence of insulin, the result is diabetes—one of the most common chronic medical conditions in industrialized countries.

Type 1 diabetes is a rare condition in which the immune system destroys the beta cells on the pancreas that make insulin. Naturally, insulin is the primary treatment for this condition, although suppressing the immune system can result in a regrowth of beta cells in some people. In type 2 diabetes, the body makes insulin, but not enough to meet the body's needs because the cells of the body are resistant to it. Fat cells are inherently resistant to insulin, so obesity is a significant risk factor for the development of type 2 diabetes. In both type 1 and type 2 diabetes, the blood glucose levels are elevated without adequate therapy and can predispose people to blindness, nerve damage, kidney damage, and cardiovascular disease.

All of the medications in this chapter should be in used in conjunction with a daily exercise and nutrition program for maximal benefit. Most of the medications in this chapter are indicated for the treatment of type 2 diabetes, which accounts for around 90 percent of total diabetes cases. *It is very important that you and your doctor know if you have pre-existing kidney disease when taking any of the diabetic medications in this chapter.*

Metformin (Glucophage) is probably the most common medication prescribed initially for diabetes, although it is not indicated if you have type 1 diabetes. While exercising and maintaining a proper diet are important in sustaining a healthy weight if you have diabetes, one of the benefits of being on this medication is that, by increasing the efficiency with which the body is able to utilize insulin, it helps to promote weight loss.

Sulfonylureas are one of the oldest medication classes for the treatment of diabetes. While potent, these are not without side effects. Commonly prescribed medications in this class include glipizide (Glucotrol®), glyburide (Micronase®), and glimepiride (Amaryl®).

Thiazolidinediones (TZDs) are a class of medications with a side-effect profile that has been publicized in the media. While an effective treatment for diabetes, it is associated with an increased risk of weight gain, heart failure, and the development of bladder cancer. Medications in this class include pioglitazone (Actos®) and rosiglitazone (Avandia®).

Incretins represent two classes of diabetes medications—the glucagon-like peptide-1 (GLP-1) agonists and dipeptidyl peptidase-4 (DPP-4) inhibitors—that work in several ways to treat diabetes, including increasing pancreatic insulin release, slowing down digestion, and decreasing hunger. **SGLT-2 inhibitors** represent a newer class of medications that inhibit the absorption of glucose in the kidney. Examples of medications in this class include canagliflozin (Invokana®), dapagliflozin (Farxiga®), and empagliflozin (Jardiance®).

Insulin has been a mainstay of treatment for diabetes for many years. It is essential for the treatment of type 1 diabetes and is added to the treatment of type 2 diabetes when other medications working together are not able to tightly control blood glucose levels. While insulin can help stabilize blood glucose levels, you'll read about why insulin can be a double-edged sword.

Metformin (Glucophage)

Metformin is the bedrock of type 2 diabetes treatment. It has also been prescribed for the treatment of other medical conditions, including metabolic syndrome and polycystic ovarian syndrome (PCOS). Metformin works by increasing the ability of the insulin to get into cells (i.e., by decreasing insulin resistance). It also works by decreasing excessive production of glucose in the liver.

1 Which (if any) dose of this medication are you currently taking?

☐ 500 mg, daily

☐ 500 mg, twice a day

☐ 1,000 mg, once a day in the morning

☐ 1,000 mg, twice a day

☐ Other: _____

- Most clinicians will begin patients at 500 mg and increase the dose over time. Diarrhea is a common side effect but is less likely to occur if this low initial dose is used and increased slowly over time.

- If someone develops diarrhea on regular metformin, there is an extra-long-lasting (XL) form of this medication that can alleviate this symptom.

2 Do you have kidney disease?

☐ Yes.

☐ No.

☐ I don't know.

- There is a slight risk that metformin could cause people with kidney disease to develop acidic blood due to lactic acidosis, which is a medical emergency. As of this writing, a man with a serum creatinine level of 1.5 mg/dL or a female with a serum creatinine level of 1.4 mg/dL should discontinue this medication, although recent studies show that this risk is minimal.

3 Are you scheduled for any procedure in which intravenous contrast dye will be given (e.g., CT scan, angiogram, or cardiac catheterization)?

☐ Yes.

☐ No.

- If you are planning to get a CT scan or a more interventional procedure such as a cardiac catheterization, your doctor will likely ask you to temporarily discontinue the medication for at least twenty-four to forty-eight hours prior to the procedure and twenty-four hours following the procedure, since these types of procedures have the potential to worsen kidney function.

4 Have you had your B_{12} level checked?

☐ Yes.

☐ No.

- A significant nutrient deficiency caused by this medication is B_{12} deficiency, which can lead to anemia, because metformin inhibits its absorption in the small intestine. If your B_{12} levels are low, you need to discuss supplementation of this important vitamin with your physician.

5 Have you experienced any of the following symptoms while taking this medication?

☐ Nausea

☐ Vomiting

☐ Diarrhea

☐ Other: _____

- The majority of side effects are gastrointestinal. For those who find these side effects intolerable, one option is to ask your physician if you can be switched to the XL (extended release) form.

- Unlike other antidiabetic medications, metformin does not cause hypoglycemia.

6 Are you taking any of the following medications that might interact with metformin?

☐ Quinolone antibiotics, including levofloxacin and ciprofloxacin

☐ Cimetidine (Tagamet)

☐ Cephalexin (Keflex®)

- The concurrent use of Tagamet or Keflex with metformin have been shown to elevate its blood levels, increasing the potential for hypoglycemia.

- The use of quinolone antibiotics can also cause hypoglycemia as a side effect, especially in conjunction with other medications that lower blood glucose levels.

Sulfonylureas

This older class of medications, made up of three "generations," works by increasing insulin released by beta cells in the pancreas. While effective at reducing blood sugar and being relatively inexpensive, they can cause dangerously low blood sugar.

1 Which (if any) of the following sulfonylurea medications have are you currently taking?

☐ Glimepiride (Amaryl)

☐ Glipizide (Glucotrol)

☐ Glyburide (Micronase)

☐ Other: _____

- It is very important that you and your doctor know if you have pre-existing kidney disease when taking any of the diabetic medications in this chapter. Many of these medications are eliminated by the kidneys, and in the setting of kidney disease, they can "hang around" in the body longer and increase the risk of developing hypoglycemia.

2 Do you drink alcohol?

☐ Yes.

☐ No.

- Don't mix sulfonylureas and alcohol. It can cause what is referred to by clinicians as a "disulfiram-like" reaction, which means you can develop significant nausea, vomiting, and abdominal pain for several hours after drinking alcohol.

- Alcohol consumption can also increase the risk of developing hypoglycemia, a life-threatening side effect of the sulfonylureas.

3 Do you have liver disease?

☐ Yes.

☐ No.

☐ I don't know.

- Liver disease can increase the risk of developing hypoglycemia with or without an antidiabetic medication. Additionally, if you have liver disease, sulfonylureas will stay in the body longer, increasing the risk of developing hypoglycemia and other potential side effects.

* * *

MEDICATION SPOTLIGHT

Sulfonylurea Alternatives

Repaglinide (Prandin®) and nateglinide (Starlix®) are shorter-acting sulfonylurea-like medications that are believed to be safer for patients with kidney or liver disease. Like the sulfonylureas, they work by increasing pancreatic production of insulin, but they are taken only with meals, diminishing the risk of hypoglycemia.

* * *

4 Have you experienced any of the following symptoms while taking this medication?

☐ Symptoms of hypoglycemia (dizziness, sweating, increased irritability)

☐ Weakness

- [ ] Confusion
- [ ] Skin rash
- [ ] Nausea
- [ ] Stomach upset
- [ ] Other: _____

- The sulfonylureas can cause significant hypoglycemia. Sometimes hypoglycemia can cause increased lethargy and even personality changes. Many of the sulfonylureas are longer-acting medications, so these symptoms may persist for several hours.

- Some of the sulfonylurea medications can also cause hyponatremia, or low sodium levels. If the sodium level is too low, it can cause weakness and confusion in some individuals.

- Some individuals may develop a skin rash, which is an allergic reaction to this class of medication.

5 Are you taking any of the following medications that might interact with sulfonylureas?

- [ ] Other diabetes medications
- [ ] Insulin
- [ ] Quinolone or sulfonamide antibiotics (e.g., Levaquin, Cipro, Bactrim)
- [ ] Fibrates for treating high blood triglyceride levels
- [ ] H_2 blockers (e.g., Tagamet)
- [ ] Fluconazole (Diflucan)

- The combination of sulfonylureas with other diabetes medications or certain antibiotics can increase the risk of developing hypoglycemia.

- Medications used to lower triglycerides or H_2 blockers and fluconazole (Diflucan) are enzymatic inhibitors that can increase the blood concentrations of sulfonylureas and their associated side effects.

- With regard to the H_2 blockers, cimetidine (Tagamet) is a potent inhibitor that can increase the blood concentrations of sulfonylureas, while ranitidine (Zantac®) is a modest inhibitor.

Thiazolidinediones (TZDs)

This class of medications helps in the treatment of diabetes by decreasing insulin resistance. It works on a specific receptor site, PPAR, and has a significant side effect profile.

1 Which (if any) of the following TZDs are you currently taking?

☐ Pioglitazone (Actos)

☐ Rosiglitazone (Avandia)

☐ Other: _____

2 What dose are you currently taking, at what frequency?

_____ mg _____ times a day.

3 Have you been ever diagnosed with congestive heart failure (CHF)?

☐ Yes.

☐ No.

• If you have this history, your doctor may choose not to prescribe this medication because it can increase the risk of developing edema and fluid overload, which you already would be at an increased risk of experiencing if you have a history of CHF. Clinically, we have always been surprised at the amount of (mostly fluid) weight that people lose when they stop taking this medication.

4 Have you experienced any of the following symptoms while taking this medication?

☐ Symptoms of hypoglycemia (dizziness, sweating, increased irritability)

☐ Shortness of breath

☐ Weight gain

☐ Other: _____

• As with other medication classes used to treat diabetes, this medication can cause hypoglycemia.

• Other symptoms associated with the side effects of increased weight gain and fluid retention include shortness of breath.

5 Which of the following medications are you taking that might interact with TZDs?

☐ Statins

☐ Acetaminophen (e.g., Tylenol)

☐ Anticonvulsants such as phenytoin (Dilantin) and valproic acid (Depakote)

☐ NSAIDs such as ibuprofen (Motrin, Advil), naproxen (Aleve), and celecoxib (Celebrex)

☐ Tetracycline antibiotics

☐ Fluconazole (Diflucan)

☐ Antipsychotics, including chlorpromazine (Thorazine®)

• TZDs can damage the liver, as detected by raised levels of certain liver enzymes, including AST and ALT. If you are taking statin medications (see chapter 2), this risk is increased.

• Given the serious potential risk of liver toxicity with statins, antiseizure medications, NSAIDs, tetracycline antibiotics, antipsychotics, and especially acetaminophen, we recommend that you minimize your use of these drugs while taking TZDs. Data is conflicting about whether the risk of liver damage is additive when the drugs are given together with TZDs.

6 If you are taking pioglitazone (Actos), how long have you been taking this medication?

☐ Six months or less

☐ Six months to one year

☐ One to two years

☐ Two years or more

• The studies seem to suggest that being on this medication for two years or more may increase the risk of developing bladder cancer. It is thought that using this medication for a shorter duration does not increase this risk, however.

7 What is your gender?

☐ Male

☐ Female

- TZDs are associated with an increased risk of bone fracture, and this risk is more significant in females. The mechanism for this risk is not known, but age does not seem to be a factor, as this risk is increased in women of all ages. While the use of TZDs is associated with bone demineralization, they do not seem to increase the risk of osteoporosis. Regardless, studies suggest that after stopping these medications for twelve months, there can be a reversal in bone loss.

SGLT-2 Inhibitors

This medication class works by increasing the amount of glucose that you lose in the urine, which lowers overall blood glucose levels.

1 Which (if any) of the following SGLT-2 inhibitors are you currently taking?

- ☐ Canagliflozin (Invokana)
- ☐ Dapagliflozin (Farxiga)
- ☐ Empagliflozin (Jardiance)
- ☐ Other: _____

2 What dose are you currently taking, at what frequency?

_____ mg _____ times a day.

3 Have you experienced any of the following symptoms while taking this medication?

- ☐ Increased urinary frequency
- ☐ Burning with urination and/or UTI
- ☐ Frequent yeast infections

- Increasing the urinary excretion of glucose also increases the amount of water in the urine, so a common side effect is needing to use the bathroom more often.

- Feeling a burning sensation with urination (also called "dysuria") can be a symptom of a urinary tract infection (UTI), another common side effect of SGLT-2 inhibitors. If you have recurrent UTIs, especially if you are elderly, speak with your doctor about possibly changing to another class of medication.

* * *

Diabetic Ketoacidosis

··

While this is a rare side effect, there is a chance that a patient may develop a condition called diabetic ketoacidosis (DKA) after starting an SGLT-2 medication. While this condition usually only affects those with type 1 diabetes, there have been rare cases of type 2 diabetes patients developing the condition after starting an SGLT-2 inhibitor.

Many of the symptoms associated with DKA are the "3Ps" initially associated with hyperglycemia: increased thirst (polydipsia), increased hunger (polyphagia), and increased urination (polyuria). Signs of a worsening condition can include abdominal pain, nausea, vomiting, increased lethargy, and/or urine that has a "fruity, sweet odor." When the blood glucose levels are very high, significant lethargy and coma-like symptoms can ensue. You should definitely call your doctor if you experience the 3Ps noted above, as these are signs that your blood glucose is too high.

* * *

4 Are you currently taking any of the following medications that might interact with SGLT-2 inhibitors?

☐ Diuretics, including hydrochlorothiazide, chlorthalidone (Hygroton), furosemide (Lasix), bumetanide (Bumex), torsemide (Demadex), spironolactone (Aldactone), and eplerenone (Inspra)

☐ Any other diabetic medications

☐ The antibiotic rifampin (Rifadin®)

• The SGLT-2 inhibitors can increase the risk of developing dehydration, especially in the elderly. Diuretics (chapter 3) also increase water loss in the urine and can worsen this side effect. If you are on any of the above medications (which many older adults are), speak with your doctor as to whether or not you should take SGLT-2 inhibitors.

• The combination of other diabetic medications with SGLT-2 inhibitors can increase the risk of developing hypoglycemia.

• Rifampin may decrease the blood levels and efficacy of the SGLT-2 inhibitors.

5 Do you have kidney disease?

□ Yes.

□ No.

□ I don't know.

- SGLT-2 inhibitors are less effective in patients with abnormal kidney function. Your kidney function should be monitored routinely if you are taking an SGLT-2 inhibitor. *If are taking any of the medications in this chapter and you have any question concerning your kidney function, do not hesitate to call your doctor.*

- Even if mild kidney disease is present, this medication class can increase the risk of dehydration and worsen the disease, and it can also lower your blood pressure. *Do not take an SGLT-2 inhibitor if you have severe kidney impairment.*

6 Are you pregnant or planning to become pregnant?

□ Yes.

□ No.

- While this medication class is not directly harmful to a developing fetus, the increased risk of UTIs, which can cause complications that harm a developing fetus, is a concern for pregnant females. If you are pregnant or thinking about becoming pregnant, you should have a frank discussion with your doctor about the potential benefit-harm ratio of SGLT-2 inhibitors during pregnancy.

Incretins

These medications, which are comprised of GLP-1 (glucagon-like peptide 1) agonists and DPP-4 (dipeptidyl peptidase 4) inhibitors, work by simulating the action of the hormone incretin. They work to lower glucose in several ways, including increasing the production of insulin with meals as well as decreasing hunger and slowing down the digestive process a little bit. While GLP-1 agonists are injected, DPP-4 inhibitors can be taken orally.

1 Which (if any) of the following incretins are you currently taking?

□ Exenatide (Byetta®)

□ Albiglutide (Tanzeum®)

☐ Liraglutide (Victoza®)

☐ Dulaglutide (Trulicity®)

☐ Sitagliptin (Januvia®)

☐ Linagliptin (Tradjenta®)

☐ Saxagliptin (Onglyza®)

☐ Other: _____

2 What dose are you currently taking, at what frequency?

_____ mg _____ times a day.

_____ mg on a weekly basis.

- Exenatide (Byetta) is an injection to be taken twice daily.
- Albiglutide (Tanzeum), liraglutide (Victoza), and dulaglutide (Trulicity) are weekly injections.
- Sitagliptin (Januvia) is usually prescribed to be taken daily, starting at 25 or 50 mg.
- Linagliptin (Tradjenta) is usually prescribed to be taken daily, starting at 5 mg.
- Saxagliptin (Onglyza) is usually prescribed to be taken daily, starting at 2.5 or 5 mg.

3 Have you experienced any of the following symptoms while taking this medication?

☐ Weight loss

☐ Getting full quickly

☐ Nausea and/or vomiting

☐ Abdominal pain

☐ Irritation at the injection site

☐ Angioedema

☐ Other: _____

- While all of the medications in this class cause weight loss, in patients on exenatide (Byetta) this effect is more pronounced.

- Many of these medications can cause nausea and vomiting as a side effect. If you experience these symptoms, stop taking the medication and call your doctor.

- Medications in this class have been associated with the development of pancreatitis. *If you develop severe abdominal pain while on any incretin, stop taking it and call your doctor as soon as possible!*

- GLP-1 agonists can cause irritation at the injection site, so it is important to rotate injection sites when taking them.

- DPP-4 inhibitors may increase the risk of developing angioedema, which is a severe allergic/anaphylactic reaction involving swelling of the tongue and airway. *If you have a history of ACE inhibitor-associated angioedema, please speak with your doctor before taking this medication.*

4 Do you have a family history of any of the following?

☐ Thyroid cancer, especially medullary

☐ An adrenal gland tumor called a "pheochromocytoma"

☐ A benign pituitary gland tumor called a "pituitary adenoma"

- Incretins can increase the risk of developing thyroid cancer, especially the medullary subtype. This association has been studied extensively in laboratories. While the effect is very uncommon, if you have any family history of the above conditions, have a discussion with your physician before starting any medications in this class.

5 Do you have normal kidney function?

☐ Yes.

☐ No.

☐ I don't know.

- As many of the medications in this class are eliminated by the body via the kidneys, patients with kidney problems may have to either adjust the dosage or stop taking incretins. The dosage of sitagliptin (Januvia), for example, can be decreased depending on your kidney function. This is an important conversation to have with your physician.

- While the effect is not very common, worsening kidney function (including kidney failure) has been reported with this medication class. This is usually caused by the side effects of nausea and vomiting, and resultant dehydration, associated with incretins.

- *We cannot stress enough that if you develop consistent nausea, vomiting, and/or abdominal pain when taking an incretin, you need to stop taking it and call your doctor immediately.*

6 **Which of the following medications are you currently taking that might interact with incretins?**

☐ Any diabetic medications

☐ ACE inhibitors

- The combination of incretins with other diabetic medications can increase the risk of hypoglycemia.

- A potential side effect of ACE inhibitors (chapter 3) is throat and tongue swelling (angioedema), and taking DPP-4 inhibitors with them further increases the risk of developing this dangerous condition. As many individuals with diabetes are also taking ACE inhibitors, it is very important to be aware of this interaction.

Insulin

While insulin is the treatment mainstay for type 1 diabetes, it is used for the treatment of type 2 diabetes when other medication classes discussed in this chapter are no longer effective at maintaining a controlled insulin level. Insulin is usually prescribed in conjunction with other diabetic medications.

1 **Which (if any) of the following forms of insulin are you currently taking?**

☐ Insulin glargine (Lantus®)

☐ Insulin detemir (Levemir®)

☐ Insulin lispro (Humalog®)

☐ Insulin aspart (Novolog®)

☐ Insulin isophane (Humulin® 70/30 or Humulin 75/25)

☐ Other: _____

- Insulin is produced by the pancreas twenty-four hours a day, seven days a week. When you eat, the pancreas increases its insulin production in response to the "glucose load" consumed. When physicians prescribe insulin, the goal is to prescribe it *physiologically*—that is, a "long-acting insulin" that is taken at set times along with a shorter-acting insulin that is taken with meals to meet the incoming glucose load.

- Insulin glargine (Lantus) and insulin detemir (Levemir) are examples of long-acting insulin: a single injection lasts twenty-four hours.

- Insulin lispro (Humalog) and insulin aspart (Novolog) are "short-acting insulins," usually prescribed to be taken with meals.

- Insulin isophane (Humulin 75/25 and 70/30) represents combination insulin regimens that contain both long-acting and short-acting insulin formulations together. These are often taken twice a day.

2 When do you check your blood glucose levels?

☐ In the morning

☐ Before breakfast

☐ Before lunch

☐ Before dinner

☐ Before bedtime

☐ Other: _____

☐ Never

- If you have been diagnosed with diabetes, you should be checking your blood glucose levels frequently, especially if you are taking any diabetic medication. If you are taking insulin, this is especially important. There is a definite risk of hypoglycemia when taking insulin medications.

3 Do you skip breakfast on a regular basis?

☐ Yes.

☐ No.

- If you are going to be on insulin or other diabetic medications, you should eat small, regular meals during the day to help you avoid hypoglycemia. Do not skip breakfast!

4 Have you experienced any of the following symptoms while taking insulin?

☐ Skin rash

☐ Lipoatrophy (localized loss of fat tissue)

☐ Symptoms of hypoglycemia (dizziness, sweating, increased irritability)

☐ Weight gain

☐ Other: _____

- It is important to rotate insulin injecting sites, as using the same site can increase the risk of developing a rash or lipoatrophy at the injection site.

- Once you start insulin, especially if you have type 2 diabetes, it can become even more difficult to lose weight, though it is not impossible. This is because insulin causes the body to behave like a bear preparing for hibernation: it wants to hold on to *everything*.

5 Do you have any kidney problems?

☐ Yes.

☐ No.

☐ I don't know.

- If you have kidney disease, your dose of insulin may need to be reduced, as compromised kidney function can increase the half-life of insulin, which in turn converts a short-acting insulin into a long-acting insulin and increases the risk of hypoglycemia.

6 Are you taking any of the following medications that might interact with insulin?

☐ Thiazolidinediones (TZDs)

☐ ACE inhibitors

☐ Fibrates

☐ Antibiotics

☐ Beta blockers

- If you are on insulin and TZDs, the effects of weight gain and fluid retention can be magnified.

- Medications that increase the hypoglycemic effects of insulin, including ACE inhibitors, fibrates, and quinolone antibiotics (Levaquin and Cipro, for example) should be used with caution by diabetes patients.

- Beta blockers can mask the symptoms of hypoglycemia (except for sweating) and prolong its duration.

Insulin—A Double-Edged Sword

If you have type 1 diabetes, you need to be on insulin because your pancreas is not making it, but if you have type 2 diabetes, your goal is to NOT be on insulin. This is because insulin is a "double-edged sword": while it allows you to control your blood glucose levels, it can make weight loss difficult. Why is this important? Because the hallmark of type 2 diabetes is insulin resistance, which usually coincides with obesity.

Think of insulin as a storage hormone—like a bear eating enough food to last through winter hibernation, insulin wants your body to store and hold on to everything. This is why it can be very difficult to lose weight when you are taking insulin, especially if you are on large doses. In fact, many people note that they gain a significant amount of weight after starting insulin.

If you are overweight and taking insulin, one of the keys to losing that excess weight is to reduce the amount of insulin you are taking. If you are able to begin an exercise program and if you change your diet to consume more plant-based and lower-glycemic foods (i.e., foods that don't stimulate a lot of insulin production), you will find that you need less insulin, helping you to lose weight.

In the beginning, these diet and lifestyle changes can be challenging, but they are not impossible. Meals should be planned in advance and prepared at home as often as possible. If you are going out to eat, study the menu ahead of time and ask questions about it. Try to substitute a vegetable for a starch. Little things like this can pay big dividends in the long run.

That being said, remember that uncontrolled high blood glucose levels increase the risk of developing complications of diabetes, including blindness and kidney disease (nephropathy). You can keep the amount of insulin you need to a minimum with the measures mentioned above, but many individuals may still need insulin even after making these diet and lifestyle changes. Whatever you do, don't avoid taking insulin if you really need it.

* * *

Notes

Notes

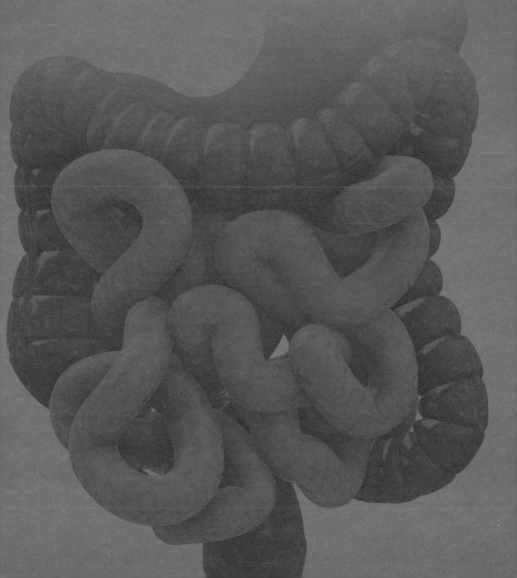

Heartburn & GI-Related Issues

Heartburn & GI-Related Issues

ONE OF THE MOST COMMON REASONS THAT PATIENTS SEE their physicians is for stomach and other gastrointestinal complaints. Medications that treat various ailments of the stomach and small intestine remain among the most commonly prescribed medications.

Histamine (H$_2$) blockers are often prescribed for the treatment of heartburn, ulcers, or other stomach upset. Medications in this class include famotidine (Pepcid®), ranitidine (Zantac), nizatidine (Axid®), and cimetidine (Tagamet). While they are often thought of as benign, these medications can have side effects such as sedation and lethargy, especially in the elderly.

Proton pump inhibitors (PPIs) are in the top ten of classes of medications most often prescribed by physicians. They are effective for the treatment of many conditions, including heartburn, ulcers, and generalized stomach upset (i.e., dyspepsia). There is no doubt that these medications are effective. They help reduce and, in many cases, completely eradicate symptoms. The big clinical question that health professionals are discussing is whether they should be restricted to short-term use, as significant side effects are associated with their long-term use.

Sucralfate (Carafate®) is an older medication used for the treatment of ulcer disease and gastritis. It works by forming a protective coating over the "injured" or ulcerated stomach area. However, it contains aluminum, which is bad for people with chronic kidney failure.

Prokinetic agents are commonly prescribed for a condition called "gastroparesis," which refers to the slowing of the movements of the small and large intestines, often resulting from diabetes. Medications prescribed for this condition include metoclopramide (Reglan®) and erythromycin, although there are certain caveats and possible side effects to watch out for.

Last but not least, various antibiotics are used for the treatment of different types of inflammation of the colon (i.e., colitis), including levofloxacin (Levaquin), ciprofloxacin (Cipro), and metronidazole (Flagyl). These will be discussed in chapter 9.

Histamine (H_2) Blockers

These medications work by inhibiting acid secretion in the stomach. While they have historically been very popular, since the advent of the PPIs they have not been prescribed as often.

1 Which (if any) of the following H_2 blockers are you currently taking?

☐ Famotidine (Pepcid)

☐ Ranitidine (Zantac)

☐ Cimetidine (Tagamet)

☐ Nizatidine (Axid)

☐ Other: _____

- Clinically, famotidine (Pepcid) and ranitidine (Zantac) are the most commonly prescribed medications of this class. They can be taken either once or twice a day.

- Tagamet is an older medication that is not as commonly prescribed. It is known as an "enzymatic inhibitor," meaning it can slow down the processing of other medications. Because of this, it can increase the risk of drug-drug interactions.

2 Why have you been prescribed this medication?

☐ Acid reflux

☐ Ulcer disease

☐ Cough that occurs only at night

☐ Allergies

☐ Other: _____

- This class of medications is most commonly prescribed to treat acid reflux and heartburn-type symptoms as well as ulcer disease.

- A cough that occurs only at night may be due to acid reflux, which may be the reason your doctor prescribed this medication. Other nonpharmacologic measures include avoiding snacks after dinner, keeping the head of the bed elevated, and losing weight.

- H_2 blockers can also be used to treat allergies as well as acute allergic reactions. They can be prescribed along with diphenhydramine (Benadryl), which is a histamine (H_1) blocker.

3 Have you experienced any of the following symptoms while taking this medication?

☐ Fatigue

☐ Drowsiness

☐ Confusion

☐ Anaphylactic reaction (swollen tongue, swelling of airway, difficulty breathing)

☐ Other: _____

- Even though these medications target H_2 receptors rather than H_1 receptors, they can cause fatigue and drowsiness, especially in the elderly population.

- H_2 blockers can cause confusion, and this risk is increased for the elderly.

- Some articles in medical peer-reviewed journals have associated anaphylaxis with ranitidine (Zantac), although this type of reaction can occur with any medication in susceptible individuals.

4 Are you taking any of the following medications that might interact with H_2 blockers?

☐ Theophylline (Theo-Dur)

☐ Warfarin (Coumadin)

☐ Benzodiazepines such as lorazepam (Ativan) or alprazolam (Xanax)

- Cimetidine (Tagamet) is an inhibitor of the CYP450 system and can decrease the metabolism of various enzymatic pathways. It is not often prescribed because it has the propensity to interact with many medications. For example, it can increase the half-life (and side effects) of both theophylline (Theo-Dur) and warfarin (Coumadin). However, *Tagamet is available over-the-counter for heartburn, so it is very important to check with your doctor or pharmacist before taking it with or without a prescription.*

- While there is no direct interaction between H_2 blockers and benzodiazepines (e.g., Ativan, Valium) per se, all of these medications can cause sedation and lethargy, especially for the elderly. The effects of these two classes of medication together can cause significant drowsiness and confusion.

Proton Pump Inhibitors (PPIs)

These popular medications, while significantly alleviating the symptoms of heartburn and peptic ulcer disease, can be associated with several potential side effects you need to be aware of. In addition to asking your doctor why you are being prescribed these medications, it is important to inquire about the length of treatment, as long-term use increases the risks of developing the side effects.

1 Which (if any) of the following PPIs are you currently taking?

☐ Lansoprazole (Prevacid®)

☐ Pantoprazole (Protonix®)

☐ Omeprazole (Prilosec®)

☐ Esomeprazole (Nexium®)

☐ Other: _____

2 What dose are you currently taking, at what frequency?

_____ mg _____ times a day.

3 Why have you been prescribed this medication?

☐ Acid reflux, including heartburn and nighttime coughing

☐ Stomach upset

☐ Peptic ulcer

☐ Gastritis

☐ Other: _____

4 How long have you been taking this medication?

☐ Less than six weeks

☐ More than six weeks

- *These medications should never be taken indefinitely.* If you have symptoms of acid reflux or stomach upset, the normal course of action is to take a PPI for six weeks and then be reassessed by the doctor to see if further investigation or treatment is needed. This is important because long-term use of PPIs is associated with certain adverse effects, including osteoporosis and bone fracture.

5 Have you experienced any of the following while taking PPIs?

☐ Bone fracture

☐ Diarrhea

☐ Weakness

☐ Fatigue

☐ Muscle twitching

☐ Other: _____

- PPIs interfere with the absorption of key bone nutrients, including calcium and vitamin C, so the risk of developing osteoporosis and/or sustaining bone fractures increases the longer you take the PPI. *It needs to be noted that the fracture risk associated with PPIs can occur in young people.*

- If you are a postmenopausal woman, taking a PPI doubles your risk for sustaining a serious fracture.

- A potential side effect of this medication is diarrhea. For some, the diarrhea can be significant enough that the medication needs to be stopped.

- Some studies demonstrate that PPIs increase the risk of developing *Clostridium difficile* colitis, a serious intestinal infection that can cause diarrhea and lead to hospitalization. Refer to the References section for more information on this.

- PPIs can interfere with the absorption of magnesium. Signs and symptoms of low magnesium levels can include weakness, fatigue, muscle twitching, and heart arrhythmias.

* * *

CONDITION SPOTLIGHT

PPI-Induced Micronutrient Deficiency

Chronic PPI use is associated with deficiencies in several key micronutrients, including calcium, magnesium, iron, vitamin C, and vitamin B_{12}. This is thought to result from the long-term suppression of stomach acid, which can interfere with the digestion of proteins and the absorption of vitamins and minerals. A complete blood count (CBC) test should be ordered before a PPI is prescribed, and a patient's magnesium, B_{12}, and iron levels should be routinely monitored while taking them. If your medical situation requires chronic use of PPIs, magnesium levels should be assessed routinely and supplemented when low.

Deficiencies of iron and B_{12} can contribute to the development of anemia. As mentioned, patients who are taking a PPI should always consult their doctors about the benefit/risk ratio of taking these medications over the long term. *If you develop symptoms such as weakness, fatigue, or muscle twitching, these may indicate anemia or a micronutrient deficiency. Please call your doctor.*

* * *

6 Are you taking any of the following medications that might interact with PPIs?

- ☐ Diuretics

- ☐ Clopidogrel (Plavix)

- ☐ Methotrexate (Rheumatrex®)

- ☐ Antifungal medications (e.g., Diflucan)

- If you have any heart-related medical issues or are taking medications that can also cause low magnesium levels (such as diuretics), you may need to supplement magnesium.

- There is a significant interaction between PPIs and clopidogrel (Plavix), an antiplatelet agent commonly prescribed by cardiologists in the wake of an acute heart attack as well as after a cardiac catheterization procedure. For many people, the simultaneous administration of Plavix and the PPI pantoprazole (Protonix), in particular, can interfere with the blood-thinning actions of Plavix by delaying its activation. The clinical significance of this interaction continues to be debated among health professionals.

- If you are taking the medication methotrexate (Rheumatrex)—which may be prescribed for cancer, psoriasis, or rheumatoid arthritis—the use of PPIs may increase its half-life, leading to very serious side effects, including liver damage.

- It is important to understand that many medications require an acidic pH environment in order to be absorbed by the body. The use of PPIs may also decrease the ability of antifungal medications to "eradicate yeast," since consistently alkaline stomach pH serves as a stimulus for continued yeast overgrowth.

Sucralfate (Carafate)

This medication, which has been around for at least two decades, is prescribed for the treatment of peptic ulcer disease. It works by forming a protective coating on the inflamed area or the ulcer.

1 What dose (if any) are you currently taking, at what frequency?

_____ mg _____ times a day.

2 Have you experienced any of the following symptoms while taking this medication?

☐ Stomach upset

☐ Nausea

☐ Vomiting

☐ Diarrhea

☐ Constipation

☐ Skin rash

☐ Other: _____

- While this medication is "GI protective," it can cause stomach upset and many GI-related symptoms noted above.

- Sucralfate (Carafate) can cause a skin rash in some individuals—a sign of an allergic reaction that may require its discontinuation.

3 Are you taking any of the following medications that might interact with Carafate?

☐ Quinolone-type antibiotics such as ciprofloxacin (Cipro) and levofloxacin (Levaquin)

☐ Tetracycline antibiotics

- You should take the above medications two hours after taking sucralfate (Carafate), as it can decrease their absorption.

4 Do you have kidney disease?

☐ Yes.

☐ No.

☐ I don't know.

- If you have moderate to severe kidney disease, sucralfate (Carafate) should be avoided because it contains aluminum, which can accumulate in the body if kidney function is not optimal.

Prokinetics

These medications are prescribed for the treatment of problems with "gastric emptying" or stomach or intestinal "motility" disorders in which food travels more slowly through the gastrointestinal tract than it should, leading to nausea, vomiting, and abdominal pain.

1 Which (if any) of the following prokinetics are you currently taking?

☐ Metoclopramide (Reglan)

☐ Erythromycin (Erythrocin)

☐ Other: _____

- Metoclopramide (Reglan) is the most common medication prescribed for this condition.

- Note that there are ongoing clinical trials studying the effectiveness of a metoclopramide nasal spray. The results so far are encouraging, although the nasal spray may be more effective in women than men.

- Erythromycin (Erythrocin) is a macrolide antibiotic that can be prescribed to treat intestinal motility syndromes, including diabetic gastroparesis. It is often prescribed in patients who do not tolerate metoclopramide (Reglan) well, although these prokinetic agents may be combined to maximize the pro-motility effect.

2 What dose are you currently taking, at what frequency?

_____ mg _____ times a day.

- Metoclopramide (Reglan) is often prescribed to be taken at least three to four times a day, with a total daily dose of 5 to 10 mg.

- Erythromycin (Erythrocin) is often only prescribed for a short period of time, as its effectiveness in treating this condition can diminish over the course of a few weeks. Doctors call this effect "tachyphylaxis."

- *Never take more than the recommended dose of metoclopramide (Reglan) or take it for more than twelve weeks. The longer you take it, the more likely you are to develop an irreversible movement disorder called "tardive dyskinesia."*

3 Have you experienced any of the following symptoms while taking this medication?

- ☐ Dizziness
- ☐ Confusion
- ☐ Lethargy
- ☐ Nausea or stomach upset
- ☐ Diarrhea
- ☐ Lip smacking, involuntary body movements, or jerking
- ☐ Other: _____

- Many of the common side effects of metoclopramide (Reglan) include dizziness, confusion, and lethargy.

- Erythromycin (Erythrocin) has the potential to cause nausea, stomach upset, and diarrhea.

- *A very common and serious side effect associated with metoclopramide (Reglan) is the neurological condition tardive dyskinesia, which can cause lip smacking, jerking, and/or other involuntary body movements. If you are experiencing any of these side effects, stop taking it and consult your doctor immediately.*

4 Are you taking any of the following medications that might interact with prokinetics?

- ☐ Antipsychotics such as haloperidol (Haldol), olanzapine (ZyPREXA), and clozapine (Clozaril)
- ☐ Levodopa (Sinemet®)
- ☐ Digoxin (Lanoxin)
- ☐ Cyclosporine (Neoral and/or SandIMMUNE®)
- ☐ Warfarin (Coumadin)
- ☐ Theophylline (Theo-Dur)
- ☐ Lovastatin (Mevacor)
- ☐ Carbamazepine (Tegretol)
- ☐ Tacrolimus (Prograf®)
- ☐ CCBs, including verapamil (Calan) and diltiazem (Cardizem)

- While all physicians are likely attuned to this, metoclopramide (Reglan) has "Parkinson-like" side effects, so this medication should not be given to anyone with this condition—especially since it can antagonize the effects of medications prescribed to treat Parkinson's, including levodopa (Sinemet).

- Both erythromycin (Erythrocin) and metoclopramide (Reglan) affect the processing of digoxin (Lanoxin) and cyclosporine (Neoral and SandIMMUNE) in the body.

- Antipsychotic medications should NOT be taken with metoclopramide (Reglan), as they can antagonize the effects of this medication.

- Erythromycin (Erythrocin) is known as an "enzymatic inhibitor," meaning that it can slow down or inhibit the processing of other medications in the liver, leading to serious side effects. For example, it is known to increase the anticoagulant effect of warfarin (Coumadin) and increase the blood levels of theophylline (Theo-Dur), lovastatin (Mevacor), simvastatin (Zocor), and digoxin (Lanoxin).

- The combination of erythromycin (Erythrocin) and lovastatin (Mevacor) or simvastatin (Zocor) can potentially lead to rhabdomyolysis, a condition in which rapid muscle breakdown causes acute damage to the kidney.

- *A serious interaction between erythromycin and certain CCBs prescribed for the treatment of hypertension or cardiac arrhythmia can potentially lead to sudden cardiac death.* Significant hypotension has also been reported with this combination.

Notes

Treating Pain

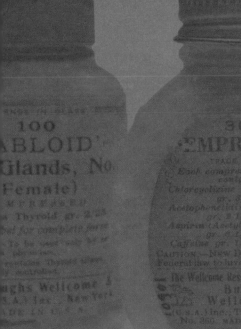
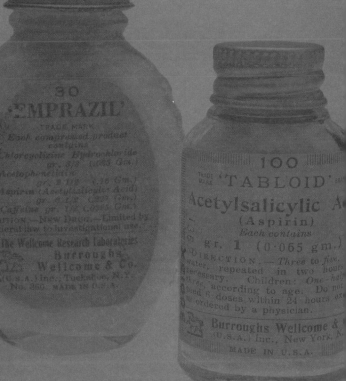

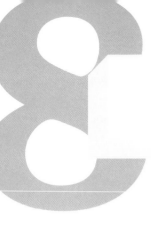

Treating
Pain

CHRONIC PAIN—ESPECIALLY BACK PAIN AND ARTHRITIS—CAN BE DEBILITATING TO the millions of people who suffer from it (particularly the elderly and those with obesity, about one out of every three in the United States). Among the most popular classes of pain medication are **aspirin** and other prescription **NSAIDs (nonsteroidal anti-inflammatory drugs)**. Common medications in this class include over-the-counter formulations of ibuprofen, including Motrin and Advil, and naproxen (Aleve). Commonly prescribed medications in this class include naproxen sodium (Naprosyn®), meloxicam (Mobic®), and celecoxib sodium (Celebrex), indomethacin (Indocin®), and diclofenac sodium (Voltaren®).

Acetaminophen (Tylenol) is the most commonly recommended medication for the treatment of pain, especially for individuals who are unable to take NSAIDs. If you have been diagnosed with any type of liver problem, however, you should speak with your doctor to see if Tylenol is right for your medical situation.

Opioids are strong-acting, narcotic pain medications that are prescribed for many types of pain, including severe arthritis when NSAIDs prove incapable of relieving the pain. While they offer effective pain relief, they are also associated with many side effects. If you have been prescribed an opioid—especially if you are elderly—be very careful. Members of this class include hydromorphone (Dilaudid®), morphine, oxycodone (OxyContin), and fentanyl (Duragesic). These medications can be prescribed orally or (in the case fentanyl) in the form of a patch. A number of opioid medications come in a combined product with acetaminophen, so you need to be careful about taking additional acetaminophen while using them.

Tramadol (Ultram) is a narcotic analgesic (painkiller) that is often prescribed by physicians as a "second-line alternative" pain treatment after NSAIDs if someone has mild to moderate pain, such as that caused by osteoarthritis.

Neuropathy medications are a range of drugs prescribed for the treatment of nerve pain. They include medications used to treat other conditions, such as depression or epilepsy, and their usefulness in treating neuropathy is considered "off-label." Examples of such medications include gabapentin (Neurontin) and amitriptyline (Elavil).

Synthetic glucocorticoids (GCs) such as prednisone (Deltasone) can be prescribed for the treatment of acute arthritic conditions, such as rheumatoid arthritis (RA) and osteoarthritis (OA), and gout. Also commonly referred to as corticosteroids, these medications are given in many forms, including injections directly into the joint and orally.

Muscle relaxants are often prescribed for the treatment of sore muscles, usually either from a sprain or strain. Their primary side effects include fatigue and sleepiness. Examples include carisoprodol (Soma®) and cyclobenzaprine (Flexeril®).

* * *

DOCTOR'S SPOTLIGHT

Polypharmacy in the Elderly

The risk of medication side effects is dramatically increased with the more medications one is taking. This is especially true for the elderly, many of whom have compromised liver or kidney function. If you are elderly, you are more likely to be dealing with chronic pain and taking several medications to treat it, including narcotics and NSAIDs, in addition to medications for a host of other diseases.

Whatever your age, you might have trouble sleeping and take a sedative such as zolpidem (Ambien) to help you get a good night's rest. You might also be on benzodiazepines such as alprazolam (Xanax) or lorazepam (Ativan) for anxiety, as you cope with rising demands in today's fast-paced world. The possible combined effects of these medications with opioids can be very dangerous.

According to a 2011 report from the National Center of Health Statistics, from 1999 to 2009 there was a dramatic increase in the number of narcotic pain medications being prescribed during that period. In 2008, "poisonings" overtook car accidents as the leading cause of accidental death. Approximately 90 percent of over forty thousand poisoning deaths that year were due to prescription medication overdoses, and opioid painkillers accounted for about 40 percent of those fatalities, followed closely by benzodiazepines, which frequently contribute to accidental deaths when taken in combination with the opioid medications.

Medications that cause drowsiness, lethargy, and/or confusion (opioids, benzodiazepines, muscle relaxants, and neuropathic pain medications) can also increase the risk of falls or car accidents, which for an elderly individual can increase the fracture risk. If you are also on warfarin (Coumadin) or other blood thinners, then in addition to the injury you sustain, you are at risk for bleeding as well.

If you have issues with chronic pain, and many of the medications discussed in this chapter are not helping at safe doses, I urge you to speak with your physician about seeing a pain management specialist. Also, note that if osteoarthritis is the source of your pain, weight reduction is a very effective strategy to reduce pain.

* * *

Aspirin

Aspirin is an anti-inflammatory medication prescribed for many health issues. This unique painkiller is believed to have heart-protective effects, and some studies suggest it may even have anticancer effects. That said, self-medicating with aspirin without first speaking with your doctor can increase your risk of developing unwanted side effects.

1 What dose do you normally take, at what frequency?

_____ mg _____ times a day.

- Common daily recommended doses of aspirin can be 81 mg, 162 mg, or 325 mg. The recommended dose depends on the reason for treatment, as well as other blood-thinning medications you may be taking. For example, if you are on warfarin (Coumadin) or another blood thinner, your doctor may choose to set your dose at 81 mg to limit the potential for bleeding complications.

- Aspirin should not be given to children without a doctor's "okay" because of the risk of Reye's syndrome, a rare but harmful disorder that can result.

* * *

CONDITION SPOTLIGHT

Salicylate Toxicity

Salicylate toxicity, which occurs when the salicylate level in the blood reaches greater than 100 mg/dL, is a medical emergency that is most commonly seen when there has been an intentional overdose of aspirin (salicylate). However, in the medical literature this has been reported to occur accidentally with the topical form of aspirin as well as when increased doses are used to treat chronic pain. Symptoms of salicylate toxicity include nausea, vomiting, tinnitus, lethargy, and hyperventilation. If the salicylate level is significantly elevated in the blood, acute dialysis may be necessary. Note that this is extremely unlikely to occur when normal doses of aspirin are taken on a daily basis.

* * *

2 Have you experienced any of the following symptoms while taking this medication?

☐ Abdominal pain

☐ Bloody stools

☐ Tinnitus (ringing in the ears)

☐ Other: _____

- Even at the above daily dosages, aspirin can increase the risk of developing problems with the stomach and small intestine, including gastritis and ulcers, which can cause bleeding from the GI (gastrointestinal) tract. If you are taking these medications, you should check your stools regularly. *If they look black or tarry or have blood in them, call your doctor right away.*

- High doses of aspirin may contribute to tinnitus.

3 Are you taking any of the following medications that might interact with aspirin?

☐ Other NSAIDs (ibuprofen [Advil], naproxen [Aleve])

☐ Platelet inhibitors (clopidogrel [Plavix], prasugrel [Effient], ticagrelor [Brilinta])

☐ Anticoagulants (apixaban [Eliquis], rivaroxaban [Xarelto], edoxaban [Savaysa], dabigatran [Pradaxa])

☐ Warfarin (Coumadin)

- The above medications increase the risk of bleeding complications when combined with aspirin, including bleeding from the GI tract.

- When combined with other NSAIDs or used in doses above 325 mg, some of aspirin's heart-protective effects are lost. If you need an antiplatelet and require high-dose chronic NSAID therapy, you may be better off on one of the above-listed antiplatelet drugs than on aspirin.

- Some people will need to take aspirin for heart protection and warfarin for atrial fibrillation, and that is okay—just look carefully for signs of bleeding.

4 Are you taking oil of wintergreen?

☐ Yes.

☐ No.

- This is a topical form of aspirin that increases the risk of side effects, including GI bleeding and tinnitus.

Nonsteroidal Anti-Inflammatory Drugs (NSAIDs)

The nature of how these medications work is really reflected in the name: by reducing inflammation they can help relieve pain from arthritis including OA, which is caused by wear and tear on the joints over time, and RA, a severe autoimmune disorder. However, these medications are also associated with a host of side effects that you should be aware of.

1 Which (if any) of the following NSAIDs do you normally take?

☐ Ibuprofen (Motrin, Advil)

☐ Celecoxib sodium (Celebrex)

☐ Meloxicam (Mobic)

☐ Naproxen (Aleve, Anaprox®)

☐ Indomethacin (Indocin)

☐ Diclofenac sodium (Voltaren)

☐ Other: _____

- *If you checked more than one box, you need to call your doctor NOW.* For example, using prescription naproxen (Aleve, Anaprox) twice a day and then going to the supermarket for additional over-the-counter ibuprofen (Motrin, Advil) is a very bad idea. This dramatically increases the risks of developing side effects.

2 What dose do you normally take, at what frequency?

_____ mg _____ times a day.

- Many NSAIDs, such as celecoxib sodium (Celebrex) and meloxicam (Mobic), can be taken once a day.

- Naproxen (Aleve, Anaprox) and indomethacin (Indocin) can be taken twice a day.

3 Have you experienced any of the following symptoms while taking this medication?

☐ Abdominal pain

☐ Bloody stools

☐ High blood pressure

☐ Edema

☐ Other: _____

- NSAIDs can increase the risk of developing problems with the stomach and small intestine, including gastritis and ulcers, which can cause bleeding from the GI tract. If you are taking these medications, you should check your stools regularly.

4 Are you taking any of the following medications that might interact with NSAIDs?

☐ ACE inhibitors

☐ ARBs

☐ Diuretics

☐ Sulfamethoxazole/trimethoprim (Bactrim)

☐ Blood thinners

- NSAIDs can cause salt and water retention and also raise blood pressure. Thus, they can antagonize the effects of medications that lower blood pressure as well as blunt the actions of diuretics.

- NSAIDs can increase the risk of bleeding from the GI tract, and this effect can be potentiated if you are taking medications that thin the blood. If you are taking any blood thinners, speak with your doctor to see if you should still be taking an NSAID.

5 Have you been diagnosed with any of the following conditions?

☐ Kidney disease

☐ High blood pressure

☐ High potassium levels

- NSAIDs can worsen kidney function and raise potassium levels. This risk increases if you are dehydrated or if you are taking medications such as ACE inhibitors, ARBs, or diuretics for high blood pressure or other cardiovascular issues. *If you are on these medications, your kidney function and potassium levels should be checked periodically, and if you develop any nausea, vomiting, diarrhea, or other acute illness, call your doctor immediately.*

- If your blood pressure is difficult to lower despite being on prescription antihypertensives, you may need to decrease or discontinue your NSAID.

Acetaminophen (Tylenol)

Acetaminophen remains one of the most commonly prescribed medications for the treatment of mild to moderate pain from arthritis or muscle soreness. It is also prescribed for lowering the body temperature if a fever is present. It is available over the counter (OTC) and in combination with other prescription and nonprescription drugs. Unlike NSAIDs, acetaminophen does not increase blood pressure or impact the heart-protective effects of aspirin.

1 What dose do you normally take, at what frequency?

_____ mg _____ times a day.

- *Do not take more than 3,500–4,000 mg a day, as more than 4,000 mg (assuming you have no prior liver problems) of a cumulative daily dose can be toxic to the liver.* Most physicians will recommend 325 mg to 650 mg, two to three times a day.

- Some people will take eight to ten acetaminophen 325 mg tablets a day (3,250 mg), along with nighttime cold relievers, opioid combination products, and other combination products that contain acetaminophen, unknowingly pushing them over the limit.

2 Do you have liver disease?

☐ Yes.

☐ No.

☐ I don't know.

- If you have liver disease, speak with your doctor about whether you should take Tylenol, and how much. Your liver may not be able to handle more than half of the standard dose.

* * *

CONDITION SPOTLIGHT

Acute Liver Failure

Tylenol is harmful to the liver because it depletes the liver cells of glutathione, which is a potent cell antioxidant. For this reason, it is dangerous to take more than the recommended daily dose. Hundreds of other prescription and nonprescription medications contain acetaminophen, so it is not uncommon for patients to be hospitalized for unintentional acute acetaminophen toxicity or overdose, which can potentially cause acute liver failure.

If you drink alcohol on a daily basis, your liver function may already be compromised, and if you are an alcoholic, taking even a small dose of Tylenol is a "double whammy" that can be toxic to your liver. Symptoms of "liver toxicity" include a yellowing of the eyes (icterus) or skin (jaundice), confusion, and fatigue.

* * *

3 How many years have you been taking Tylenol on a steady basis?

☐ Less than five years

☐ Five to ten years

☐ More than ten years

- There have been reports of chronic Tylenol use (taken more days than not) over many years affecting the kidneys.

4 Are you taking any of the following medications that might contribute to acetaminophen overdose?

☐ Oxycodone/acetaminophen (Percocet®)

☐ Hydrocodone/acetaminophen (Vicodin®)

☐ Acetaminophen/aspirin/caffeine (Excedrin®)

☐ Other acetaminophen-containing OTC medications for pain, cold, sinus, or cough

- Oxycodone/acetaminophen (Percocet) and hydrocodone/acetaminophen (Vicodin) are prescription pain medications that contain acetaminophen. As discussed above, too much of this medication can be very harmful to your liver. *If you are taking these prescription medications, please do not take Tylenol at the same time.*

- Hundreds of OTC formulations intended for the treatment of pain or of cold and cough symptoms—including such popular brands as DayQuil®, Dimetapp®, Excedrin, Midol®, NyQuil, Robitussin, Sudafed®, Theraflu®, and Vicks®—contain acetaminophen. If you are taking one or more of these, or if you have been prescribed an acetaminophen-containing drug such as Vicodin, it is very important to read the labels on all medications indicated for the treatment of pain, cold, and cough, so you can make sure you are not taking more than the daily recommended dose.

Opioids

Opioids are narcotic medications derived from opium and its painkilling alkaloid, morphine. They are often prescribed for the treatment of chronic pain when other non-narcotic painkillers, such as NSAIDs and acetaminophen, are not effective enough. *However, because of their euphoric effects, they have high addictive potential, and their sedative properties make them dangerous when taken in high doses or in combination with other sedating medications or substances, including alcohol.*

1 Which (if any) of the following opioids are you currently taking?

☐ Morphine

☐ Hydromorphone (Dilaudid)

☐ Oxycodone (OxyContin)

☐ Hydrocodone/acetaminophen (Vicodin)

☐ Oxycodone/acetaminophen (Percocet)

☐ Other: _____

- If you are taking more than one medication listed above, talk to your doctor to make sure that this is okay. Sometimes it may be warranted—for example, a physician might prescribe a longer-acting narcotic along with a shorter-acting narcotic to cancer patients to treat breakthrough pain. However, two shorter-acting narcotics are not a good combination.

2 What dose are you currently taking, at what frequency?

_____ mg _____ times a day.

3 Have you experienced any of the following symptoms while taking this medication?

☐ Constipation

☐ Confusion

☐ Dizziness

☐ Drowsiness

☐ Lethargy

☐ Other: _____

- Constipation as a significant side effect of opioids. If you are prescribed a narcotic pain medication, your doctor may also prescribe a stool softener like docusate (Colace®) or a natural laxative such as senna (Senokot®).

- Opioids can cause confusion, especially in the elderly.

- Opioids are also known to cause significant drowsiness, especially at higher doses and in the elderly.

* * *

Opioid Overdose

In addition to lethargy, a significant possible side effect is depression of the respiratory drive. You need to be especially mindful of this if you are elderly, if you have an underlying lung problem such as emphysema or asthma, or if you are on other medications, such as sleep aids or antianxiety agents, that can also have a sedating effect.

Signs of overdose include increased lethargy, slurred speech, and breathing at a much slower rate than normal. This can be potentially fatal, especially if left undiagnosed. *If a loved one is exhibiting any of the above symptoms, do not leave him or her alone. Call 911 immediately.* The Emergency Medical Services (EMS) personnel will likely emergently prescribe naloxone (Narcan®), an opioid antagonist that can be lifesaving.

The laws in many states are changing to allow family members of people who are opioid dependent or addicted to opioids to administer naxolone to their loved ones. You will need special training before administering the drug, however.

* * *

4 Are you taking any of the following medications or substances that might interact with opioid painkillers?

☐ SSRIs

☐ Tricyclic antidepressants

☐ Antihistamines such as diphenhydramine (Benadryl)

☐ Muscle relaxants

☐ Antipsychotics

☐ Sleep aids

☐ Alcohol

- Hydrocodone/acetaminophen (Vicodin) and oxycodone (OxyContin) are in part metabolized by the CYP2D6 pathway, as are certain anti-depressants. Some antidepressants and diphenhydramine can also inhibit processing in this pathway, which may decrease the analgesic effects of these opioids and increase the risk of developing possible side effects or even serotonin syndrome (see chapter 5).

- Please refer to chapter 5 to review the potentially dangerous interactions between opioids and various sedating medications.

- *Do not drink alcohol if you are on an opioid. Alcohol is a depressant of the respiratory drive and can stop someone from breathing if used with opioids.*

Tramadol (Ultram)

This is a narcotic medication that is often prescribed by physicians for the treatment of chronic pain, especially due to arthritis, of those for whom NSAIDs are ineffective or not well tolerated.

1 Are you currently taking tramadol (Ultram)?

☐ Yes.

☐ No.

2 What dose are you currently taking, at what frequency?

_____ mg _____ times a day.

- This medication is commonly dosed to be taken 50 mg every six hours. There is also an extended-release form of this medication.

3 Have you experienced any of the following symptoms while taking this medication?

☐ Lethargy

☐ Drowsiness

☐ Confusion

☐ Dizziness

☐ Headache

☐ Nausea

☐ Other: _____

- Tramadol is a narcotic analgesic that can cause many of the sedating side effects of the other opioid medications, including lethargy, drowsiness, and confusion.

4 **Are you taking any of the following medications that might interact with tramadol (Ultram)?**

☐ SSRIs

☐ Tricyclic antidepressants

☐ Antihistamines such as diphenhydramine (Benadryl)

☐ Antiseizure medications

☐ Antipsychotics

☐ Sleep aids

- Tramadol (Ultram) is metabolized by the CYP2D6 pathway and also acts on serotonin receptors as an SNRI. If you are also on antidepressants such as SSRIs, many of which inhibit this pathway, you risk the development of serotonin syndrome (see chapter 5 for more information on major drug-drug interactions that can lead to this serious condition). *If you experience such symptoms as increased heart rate, muscle twitching, and high body temperature (hyperthermia), get help immediately.*

- Be careful if you are taking this medication in conjunction with opioids or sedating medications.

Neuropathy Medications

Neuropathy and nerve pain can be particularly disabling, affecting one's ability to walk. While there can be many causes of nerve pain, three of the most common causes that doctors see are pain due to back problems caused by severe degenerative arthritis, spinal stenosis, or herniated discs; neuropathy related to diabetes; and nerve pain accompanying a shingles outbreak (postherpetic neuralgia).

1 **Which (if any) of the following medications are you currently taking?**

☐ Nortriptyline (Pamelor)

☐ Amitriptyline (Elavil)

☐ Valproic acid (Depakote)

☐ Gabapentin (Neurontin)

☐ Pregabalin (Lyrica®)

☐ Duloxetine (Cymbalta)

☐ Other: _____

- Nortriptyline (Pamelor) and amitriptyline (Elavil) are examples of "tricyclic antidepressants." In addition to treating depression, they can be effective in the treatment of chronic pain.

- Valproic acid (Depakote) and gabapentin (Neurontin) are used to treat seizures, and Depakote is also used to treat migraine headaches.

- Pregabalin (Lyrica) is FDA-approved for the treatment of fibromyalgia, but it has been used for the treatment of nerve pain as well.

2 What dose are you currently taking, at what frequency?

_____ mg _____ times a day.

3 Have you experienced any of the following symptoms while taking this medication?

☐ Confusion

☐ Lethargy

☐ Urinary retention

☐ Dizziness when standing up

☐ Slow heart rate

☐ Twitching

☐ Other: _____

- All of the above medications can cause confusion and lethargy, especially in the elderly.

- Nortriptyline (Pamelor) and amitriptyline (Elavil) can cause urinary retention and dizziness when standing up.

- Gabapentin (Neurontin) can cause twitching in some people.

4 Have you been diagnosed with any of the following conditions?

☐ Kidney disease

☐ Liver disease

☐ Glaucoma

- If you have kidney disease, then the dose of gabapentin (Neurontin) should be increased slowly from a low starting dose.

- Valproic acid (Depakote) can affect liver function. If you are taking this medication, your doctor should be ordering blood tests to track your liver enzyme levels.

- Although neuropathy medications are not directly toxic to the liver or kidneys, starting doses may need to be reduced if you have liver or kidney disease. Liver and kidney function should be periodically monitored as well.

- Tricyclic antidepressants can worsen glaucoma, so if you have been diagnosed with this condition, check with your doctor about other options for treating nerve pain.

Synthetic Glucocorticoids (GCs)

Synthetic glucocorticoids are steroid medications that treat chronic pain associated with many arthritic conditions by reducing inflammation. That being said, they are associated with a host of side effects and should be taken with caution.

1 Which (if any) of the following GCs are you currently taking?

☐ Prednisone (Deltasone)

☐ Hydrocortisone (Cortef®)

☐ Methylprednisolone (Medrol Dosepak®)

☐ Other: _____

- Prednisone (Deltasone) is the most common type of steroid prescribed for pain and inflammation.

2 What dose are you currently taking, at what frequency?

_____ mg _____ times a day.

- GCs are often dosed to be decreased slowly over time, since stopping this medication cold turkey may have dire consequences. Your adrenal glands produce cortisol, a natural steroid, so when you take a synthetic steroid—especially doses higher than 10 mg daily—the action of your adrenal glands may be suppressed. *Do not suddenly stop taking this medication without talking to your doctor first.*

MEDICATION SPOTLIGHT

GC Injections and Inhalants

There is more than one way to take a GC. Doctors can inject it directly into a joint, to treat joint pain caused by painful gout or osteoarthritis, for example. GCs can be injected into the back for the treatment of back pain or given as an inhalant for the acute and chronic treatment of problems such as asthma and emphysema. The advantage of a localized injection is that absorption into the bloodstream is lessened, reducing the likelihood of certain side effects. Inhalants and local injections may still have a mild systemic effect, reducing overall inflammation but also raising blood pressure and blood glucose levels, although the effect is not as strong as that caused by pills or injections into the blood.

* * *

3 Have you experienced any of the following symptoms while taking this medication?

- ☐ High blood pressure
- ☐ Leg swelling
- ☐ Psychotic behavior
- ☐ Increased appetite
- ☐ Weight gain
- ☐ Infection
- ☐ Insomnia
- ☐ Other: _____

- Prednisone (Deltasone) can raise blood pressure and cause leg swelling.

- When some people take prednisone (Deltasone), they develop psychotic behavior, known as "steroid psychosis." This can occur even at low doses of prednisone—i.e., 5–10 mg—in some cases.

- Many people on synthetic steroids will notice a marked increase in appetite and weight gain, especially if they are taking them for a few weeks.

- It is important to know that when you are on GCs, your immune system is compromised, and this can make you more susceptible to infection.

- A common side effect of GCs is trouble sleeping and insomnia.

4 Have you ever been diagnosed with either of the following conditions?

☐ Osteoporosis

☐ Diabetes

- Synthetic steroids can increase the risk of developing osteoporosis. After someone has been on steroids for as little as three to four weeks, changes in bone density may result.

- Many doctors will order a dual-energy absorptiometry scan (DXA) if you are going to be on steroids for more than a couple of weeks.

- You should take calcium and vitamin D supplements during your GC treatment.

- Steroids can also raise blood glucose levels, and in some patients they may be associated with the development of diabetes.

5 Are you also taking an NSAID in addition to your GC?

☐ Yes.

☐ No.

- When used on their own, GCs can cause stomach upset and can increase the chance of developing gastritis and ulcer disease. Taking an NSAID in addition to a GC increases the risk of developing stomach problems. If you are taking an NSAID of any type (even OTC medications such as Motrin or Advil), speak with your doctor about whether these medications should be avoided while you are on prednisone or another GC.

- Many health-care professionals may also prescribe "stomach protectors," such as H_2 blockers and PPIs, to help protect against stomach-related ailments.

Muscle Relaxants

Muscle pain, spasms, and inflammation can often accompany arthritis pain or occur on their own. These medications reduce pain by suppressing muscle spasms.

1 Which (if any) of the following muscle relaxants are you currently taking?

☐ Carisoprodol (Soma)

☐ Cyclobenzaprine (Flexeril)

☐ Methocarbamol (Robaxin®)

☐ Metaxalone (Skelaxin®)

☐ Other: _____

2 What dose are you currently taking, at what frequency?
_____ mg _____ times a day.

3 Have you experienced any of the following symptoms while taking this medication?

☐ Fatigue

☐ Confusion

☐ Lethargy

☐ Feeling "hung over" in the morning

☐ Irregular or fast heartbeat

☐ Other: _____

- Muscle relaxants are associated with many side effects, including fatigue, confusion, and increased lethargy.

- Cyclobenzaprine (Flexeril) can increase the risk of cardiac arrhythmia (irregular beating of the heart), so speak with your doctor if you have any history of heart problems.

- Many times, muscle relaxants are prescribed along with other pain medications, which can increase the risk of developing side effects.

4 Are you taking any of the following medications that might interact with muscle relaxants?

☐ SSRIs

☐ Opioid painkillers

☐ Benzodiazepines

- There have been two case reports of metaxalone (Skelaxin) causing serotonin syndrome when combined with an SSRI.

- Opioids and benzodiazepines can increase the risk of developing fatigue and lethargy when in combination with muscle relaxants.

Notes

Notes

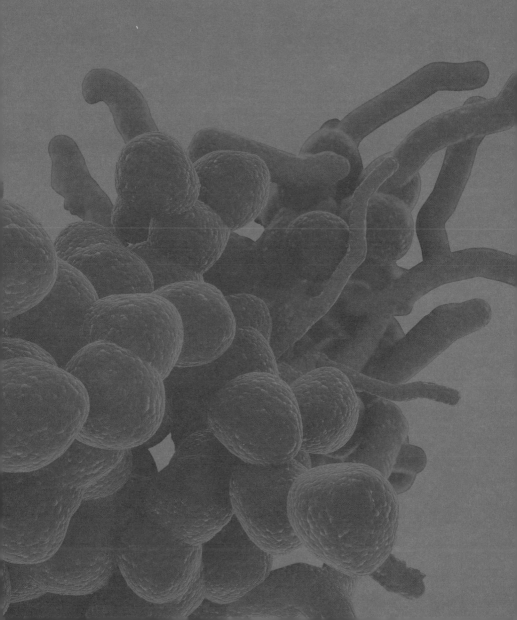

CHECKLIST 9

Antibiotics

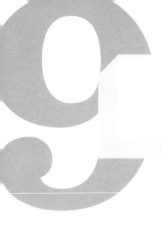

Antibiotics

MILLIONS OF ANTIBIOTICS ARE PRESCRIBED ANNUALLY BY HEALTH-CARE PROFESSIONALS. In the last several chapters, we have made reference to different antibiotics as well as interactions and side effects. In this chapter we will talk about antibiotics commonly prescribed both in the hospital and for home use.

Penicillins are one of the oldest classes of antibiotics around. They are commonly prescribed for the treatment of many types of infections, including a sore throat (pharyngitis), ear infections (otitis media), and bronchitis. Examples of penicillins commonly prescribed include amoxicillin (Amoxil®) and amoxicillin/clavulanate potassium (Augmentin®).

Macrolides are a popular group of antibiotics that have many significant drug-drug interactions. They are prescribed for a spectrum of conditions, including sinusitis and pneumonia. Medications in this class include erythromycin (Erythrocin®), clarithromycin (Biaxin), and azithromycin (Zithromax).

Cephalosporins are a close relative of the penicillins. They are made up of five "generations" of antibiotics that collectively combat a very wide range of bacteria. Medications in this class are commonly prescribed for upper respiratory infections (URIs), pneumonia, and skin infections such as cellulitis, although they are also utilized for the treatment of sexually transmitted infections, meningitis, and hospital-acquired infections. Examples include cefazolin (Ancef®) and cefpodoxime (Vantin®).

Quinolones are commonly prescribed for the treatment of urinary tract infections (UTIs) and lung infections, especially pneumonia. They may also be prescribed for skin infections. Examples of medications in this class are ciprofloxacin (Cipro) and levofloxacin (Levaquin).

Sulfamethoxazole/trimethoprim (Bactrim) is the most commonly prescribed of the sulfonamide antibiotics. It is usually used for lung infections and UTIs.

Penicillins

Penicillins are widely prescribed for ear, throat, and lung infections. Although they are considered a first-line treatment for many types of infections, not everyone can tolerate them.

1 Which (if any) of the following penicillins are you currently taking?

☐ Amoxicillin (Amoxil, Trimox®)

☐ Amoxicillin/clavulanate potassium (Augmentin)

☐ Other: _____

2 Do you have a penicillin allergy?

☐ Yes.

☐ No.

☐ I don't know.

- If you have a penicillin allergy, it is important to tell your doctor. If you have had a true documented allergic reaction—i.e., hives, skin rash, and/or swelling of the tongue—then you should not be taking this class of medication. If your reaction was "stomach upset," then it is probably not a true allergy.

- Given the increase in bacterial resistance to many antibiotics across the board, if you have an infection and your doctor is able to prescribe you penicillin, he or she will.

3 Why have you been prescribed this medication?

☐ UTI

☐ Sinus infection

☐ Pharyngitis

☐ Ear infection

☐ Other: _____

- Amoxicillin (Amoxil, Trimox) or amoxicillin/clavulanate potassium (Augmentin) may be prescribed for a UTI.

- Amoxicillin (Amoxil, Trimox) is also used for the treatment of bacterial sinus infections and ear infections (otitis media).

- Penicillins are usually first-line treatments for pharyngitis, which is usually caused by strep. If you have strep but are allergic to penicillin, the next recommended antibiotic is erythromycin (Erythrocin).

4 What dose are you currently taking, at what frequency?

_____ mg _____ times a day.

- The most common dosing regimens for amoxicillin/clavulanate potassium (Augmentin) and amoxicillin (Amoxil, Trimox) are 250 mg or 500 mg, two to three times a day, for a period of a week to ten days. If there is moderate kidney dysfunction present, this dosage can be decreased to twice a day, and in the case of severe kidney dysfunction, these antibiotics will be often be dosed once a day.

5 Have you experienced any of the following symptoms while taking this medication?

☐ Nausea

☐ Vomiting

☐ Stomach upset

☐ Diarrhea

☐ Skin rash/hives

☐ Fever

☐ Tongue swelling

☐ Other: _____

- Common reactions to antibiotics include nausea, vomiting, and stomach upset.

- If you are on an antibiotic and you experience diarrhea, call your doctor and have a conversation about whether the antibiotic needs to be discontinued. Your diarrhea may be either an uncomfortable but not terribly serious side effect or a symptom of the more serious *Clostridium difficile* colitis.

- Skin rash and fever can occur with many antibiotic classes, but again, call your doctor if you experience these symptoms, as they may be early signs of an allergic reaction.

- Penicillins, as well as many other antibiotic classes, can cause severe swelling of the tongue and airway (anaphylaxis), which is life-threatening. If this ever happens to you, it is not safe for you to take any penicillin in the future.

Understanding Clostridium Difficile *Colitis*

Clostridium difficile colitis is the most common infection that occurs during a stay in the hospital, and one of the significant contributing factors to this is the overuse of antibiotics. Especially if given in multiple doses, antibiotics can affect the integrity of your bowel flora, potentially causing increased growth of a "bad bacterium" called *Clostridium difficile.* While any antibiotic can increase the risk of developing this condition, clindamycin (Cleocin®) and quinolones such as levofloxacin (Levaquin) are particularly associated with the development of this condition.

In worst-case scenarios, this type of colitis can require (further) hospitalization or even be fatal. Luckily, however, certain antibiotics may actually be prescribed for the treatment of this condition, including vancomycin (Vancocin®) and metronidazole (Flagyl).

One recommendation for preventing this type of colitis is to minimize antibiotic use, but patients can also take a probiotic with any antibiotic prescription to minimize the risk of developing this condition. Please refer to chapter 10 regarding the uses and benefits of probiotic supplementation.

* * *

6 Are you taking any of the following medications that might interact with penicillins?

☐ Warfarin

☐ Allopurinol (Zyloprim®)

☐ Methotrexate (Rheumatrex)

☐ Oral contraceptives

- The combination of amoxicillin/clavulanate potassium (Augmentin) and warfarin (Coumadin) may increase the levels of warfarin in the blood

- If you are on allopurinol (Zyloprim) and amoxicillin (Trimox), there is an increased risk for the development of a skin rash.

- Penicillins can increase the blood levels of the immunosuppressant anticancer drug methotrexate (Rheumatrex), which can potentially lead to very serious consequences.

- There have been reported cases of penicillins and other antibiotics decreasing the efficacy of the oral contraceptives in preventing pregnancy.

Macrolides

Erythromycin (Erythrocin), azithromycin (Zithromax), and clarithromycin (Biaxin) are in the group of antibiotics known as the "macrolides." They are commonly used for the treatment of UTIs, sinusitis, pharyngitis, bronchitis, and pneumonia.

1 Which (if any) of the following macrolides are you currently taking?

☐ Erythromycin (Erythrocin)

☐ Azithromycin (Zithromax)

☐ Clarithromycin (Biaxin)

☐ Other: _____

2 What dose are you currently taking, at what frequency?

_____ mg _____ times a day.

3 Have you experienced any of the following symptoms while taking this medication?

☐ Nausea

☐ Vomiting

☐ Stomach upset

☐ Diarrhea

☐ Dizziness

☐ Other: _____

- Nausea, vomiting, and stomach upset are common side effects of these medications—especially erythromycin (Erythrocin) and clarithromycin (Biaxin). Azithromycin (Zithromax) has significantly fewer GI side effects and may be an acceptable alternative if GI upset becomes intolerable.

- *If you are experiencing dizziness or lightheadedness, it is important to let your physician know.* This is because these medications can cause QT interval prolongation—a heart condition that can increase your chances of developing a cardiac arrhythmia. This can be observed on an electrocardiogram (ECG), so your doctor may need to order one. If you have any significant heart problems, your doctor will likely choose another medication.

4 Are you taking any of the following medications that might interact with macrolides?

☐ CCBs including amlodipine (Norvasc) and diltiazem (Cardizem)

☐ Statins such as simvastatin (Zocor,) atorvastatin (Lipitor), and lovastatin (Mevaco)r

- Clarithromycin (Biaxin) and erythromycin (Erythrocin) inhibit the CYP3A4 pathway in the liver, so they can inhibit the processing of other medications that are metabolized by this pathway, such as calcium channel blockers and statins like simvastatin (Zocor), lova statin (Mevacor), and atorvastatin (Lipitor). The interaction with atorvastatin is not believed to be as clinically significant as with the other two statins mentioned, although peer-reference articles mention all three.

- The drug interaction between clarithromycin (Biaxin) and CCBs is especially serious because the half-life of CCBs is extended so much that it can cause low blood pressure, which in turn can cause acute injury to the kidneys.

- Azithromycin (Zithromax) does not inhibit the CYP3A4 pathway or seem to have any significant drug-drug interactions noted above.

- As a quick reminder, simvastatin (Zocor), atorvastatin (Lipitor), and lovastatin (Mevacor) are processed by the CYP3A4 pathway in the liver. Rosuvastatin (Crestor) and pravastatin (Pravachol) are not, and therefore are safer alternatives than other statins if you are on one of these drugs and must take erythromycin (Erythrocin) or clarithro-mycin (Biaxin) for any reason. Again, note that this interaction with atorvastatin (Lipitor) is not considered to be as clinically significant as with the other two statins.

Cephalosporins

Cephalosporins, like penicillins, are known as β-lactam antibiotics. They are most commonly prescribed for skin infections but have a very wide range of potential uses.

1 Which (if any) of the following cephalosporins are you currently taking?

☐ Cephalexin (Keflex)

☐ Cefazolin (Ancef)

☐ Cefaclor (Distaclor®)

☐ Cefpodoxime (Vantin)

☐ Ceftriaxone (Rocephin®)

☐ Other: _____

2 What dose are you currently taking, at what frequency?

_____ mg _____ times a day.

- Cephalexin (Keflex) is commonly dosed at 500 mg, three to four times a day, but the dosage needs to be reduced if there is kidney dysfunction present.

3 Why have you been prescribed this medication?

☐ Skin infection (cellulitis)

☐ URI

☐ Pharyngitis

☐ Lung infection

☐ Other: _____

- Cephalexin (Keflex) is commonly prescribed for skin infections, especially cellulitis, and is taken orally, whereas cefazolin (Ancef) is the intravenous equivalent and is commonly prescribed in a hospital setting.

- Cefaclor (Distaclor) and cefpodoxime (Vantin) are often prescribed for the treatment of a URI, including sinusitis.

- Ceftriaxone (Rocephin) is a common medication given intravenously for the treatment of pneumonia.

4 Do you have a penicillin allergy?

☐ Yes.

☐ No.

☐ I don't know.

- If you have a true penicillin allergy, you have a 5 percent chance of having an allergy to cephalosporins as well. This is why physicians are very reluctant to prescribe a cephalosporin to someone with a penicillin allergy, unless the patient has taken one in the past without a problem, or there is no other reasonable antibiotic option available.

5 Have you experienced any of the following symptoms while taking this medication?

☐ Nausea

☐ Vomiting

☐ Diarrhea

☐ Stomach upset

☐ Skin rash/hives

☐ Other: _____

- The side effects associated with cephalosporins are similar to those associated with penicillins and many other types of antibiotics.

6 Which of the following medications are you currently taking that might interact with cephalosporins?

☐ Metformin

☐ Warfarin

☐ Other: _____

- Certain cephalosporins, including cephalexin (Keflex), may decrease the renal elimination of metformin (Glucophage). This interaction needs to be especially considered in patients with mild kidney disease.

- Cephalosporins may affect the metabolism of warfarin in several different ways. Patients taking both warfarin (Coumadin) and a cephalosporin will have to have their INR (international normalized ratio) levels monitored closely, and the dose of warfarin may need to be reduced.

* * *

MEDICATION SPOTLIGHT

Clindamycin

Clindamycin (Cleocin) can treat multiple types of organisms, including *Staphylococcus*, *Streptococcus*, and anaerobic types of infections. It is often used for really bad and aggressive skin infections, but physicians will also prescribe it for aspiration pneumonia. Common oral doses are 300–600 mg, three times a day, and common side effects include nausea, vomiting, and stomach upset, as with most antibiotics. One of the most frequent unintended consequences of taking clindamycin, however, is the development of *Clostridium difficile* colitis. Because of this, physicians ask patients to closely monitor for diarrhea, which could be a sign of this potentially life-threatening infection.

* * *

Quinolones

The quinolones—effective against many serious infections, including kidney infections and pneumonia—have a range of potential side effects and interactions with other prescription medications.

1 Which (if any) of the following quinolones are you currently taking?

☐ Ciprofloxacin (Cipro)

☐ Levofloxacin (Levaquin)

☐ Norfloxacin (Noroxin®)

☐ Other: _____

2 Why have you been prescribed this medication?

☐ UTI

☐ Pneumonia

☐ Colitis

☐ URI

☐ Other: _____

- Often doctors will prescribe ciprofloxacin (Cipro) or levofloxacin (Levaquin) in combination with metronidazole (Flagyl) for colitis.

3 What dose are you currently taking, at what frequency?

_____ mg _____ times a day.

- Levofloxacin (Levaquin) is prescribed to be taken once daily, usually in doses of 250 or 500 mg. There is a 750 mg dose for really bad pneumonia. If there is advanced kidney disease present, levofloxacin (Levaquin) is often prescribed every other day.

- Ciprofloxacin (Cipro) is often prescribed 250–500 mg twice daily. If kidney dysfunction is present, this medication is decreased to 250 mg, usually once a day.

- The consumption of dairy products should be restricted if quinolones (especially Cipro) are prescribed. The calcium and the protein (casein) in milk and other dairy products can decrease the absorption of these antibiotics.

4 Have you been diagnosed with any of the following conditions?

☐ Kidney disease

☐ A seizure disorder such as epilepsy

☐ Any heart-related conditions

☐ Diabetes

☐ Arthritis or asthma

- Quinolone dosage needs to be reduced if kidney disease is present.

- If you have a history of seizures, these medications can lower the seizure threshold, increasing your risk of having another.

- Quinolones can cause QT interval prolongation, which increases your chances of developing a cardiac arrhythmia. If you have any significant heart problems, your doctor will likely choose another medication.

- These medications can also cause hypoglycemia. If you have diabetes, quinolones may not be the best medications for you.

- If you are taking GCs for arthritis or asthma, there is increased risk of developing tendon rupture with quinolones.

5 Have you experienced any of the following symptoms while taking this medication?

☐ Nausea, vomiting, and/or diarrhea

☐ Leg pain and/or difficulty walking

☐ Joint pain or muscle pain

☐ Dizziness

☐ Skin rash

☐ Swelling of the tongue or throat

☐ Numbness and tingling of the hands or feet

☐ Other: _____

- In the adults and the elderly, there have been reports of rupture of the Achilles tendon caused by quinolones. This can show up as leg pain and difficulty with walking.

- Many antibiotics can cause skin rash and severe swelling of the tongue and airway (anaphylaxis), which is life-threatening. *If you experience these symptoms, call 911 immediately.*

- In addition to increased risk of tendonitis and tendon ruptures, there have been several reported cases of peripheral neuropathy with use of quinolones. Symptoms of this can include numbness and tingling in the hands and feet. *If you experience any of these symptoms while taking quinolones, stop taking the medication and call you doctor immediately.*

6 Are you taking any of the following medications that might interact with quinolones?

- ☐ Warfarin (Coumadin)

- ☐ Theophylline (Theo-Dur)

- ☐ Sucralfate (Carafate) and/or other antacids

- ☐ Diabetes-related medications

- ☐ Macrolides

- ☐ Tricyclics

- ☐ Anti-arrhythmic medications

- Quinolones interact significantly with warfarin (Coumadin), so if you are taking it, you will probably need to decrease your dose and follow your PT/INR values closely.

- Theophylline (Theo-Dur) is an older medication commonly prescribed for the treatment of asthma and emphysema. Quinolones can decrease the clearance of this medication, resulting in serious side effects, including seizures and palpitations.

- Sucralfate (Carafate), used for the treatment of peptic ulcer disease and gastritis, can decrease the absorption of quinolones. In addition, any antacid containing aluminum, calcium, and/or magnesium should be avoided, as they can also inhibit their absorption.

- As mentioned in chapter 6, the simultaneous use of quinolones and diabetes medications can increase the risk of hypoglycemia.

- Quinolones should probably be avoided if you are taking any tricyclic antidepressants, macrolide antibiotics, and/or certain anti-arrhythmic medications, since the combination may increase the risk of developing QT interval prolongation, which in turn can cause cardiac arrhythmias.

Sulfamethoxazole/trimethoprim (Bactrim)

Bactrim consists of one part trimethoprim and five parts sulfamethoxizole. It is primarily used for the treatment of UTIs but may also treat conditions such as MRSA skin infections, URIs, and traveler's diarrhea.

1 Which (if any) of the following dosages are you currently taking?

☐ Bactrim SS (single strength, 80/400)

☐ Bactrim DS (double strength, 160/800)

- The double-strength dose is often prescribed for the treatment of conditions such as UTI and URI.

2 Why have you been prescribed this medication?

☐ UTI

☐ Pneumonia

☐ URI

☐ Other: _____

- For the treatment of a simple UTI, Bactrim DS is recommended to be taken twice a day for three days. For other types of infections, including bronchitis, the duration of therapy is often ten days to two weeks.

3 Do you have a sulfa allergy?

☐ Yes.

☐ No.

☐ I don't know.

- Bactrim is a sulfa antibiotic, so if you have a sulfa allergy, you should not take it.

4 Do you have kidney disease?

☐ Yes.

☐ No.

☐ I don't know.

- If your kidney function is less than 30 percent, you should probably not be given this medication.

- Bactrim may cause an elevation in the creatinine level that may not be reflective of worsening kidney function.

5 Have you experienced any of the following symptoms while taking this medication?

☐ Nausea, vomiting, and/or diarrhea

☐ Skin rash

☐ Fever

☐ Other: _____

- The side effects associated with Bactrim are similar to those associated with many other antibiotics.

6 Are you taking any of the following medications that might interact with Bactrim?

☐ Heart or blood pressure medications, including ACE inhibitors and ARBs

☐ Diuretics

☐ NSAIDs

☐ Warfarin

- Bactrim can cause high potassium levels (hyperkalemia), so if you are on heart or blood pressure medications that can also raise potassium levels (e.g., ACE inhibitors, ARBs, diuretics) and/or on NSAID pain medications, you need to have your kidney function and potassium levels monitored.

- If you are taking Bactrim and warfarin (Coumadin), you may need to have your warfarin dosing and INR monitored closely, as there have been reports of increased bleeding risk with this drug combination.

Notes

Notes

Natural
Supplements

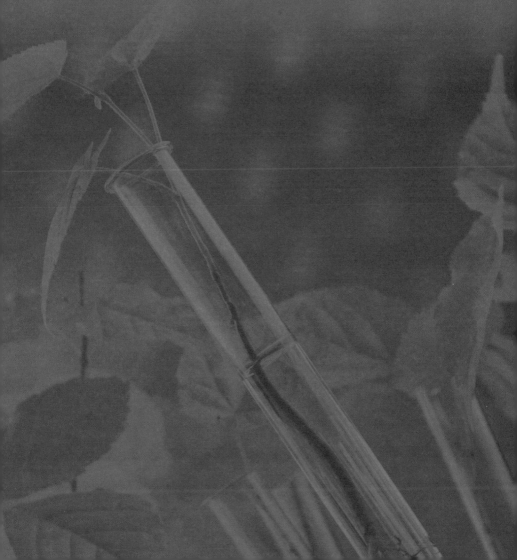

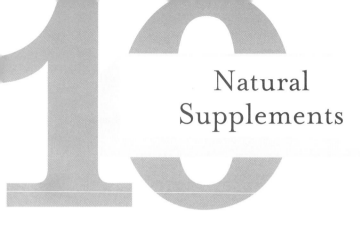

Natural
Supplements

MORE THAN 62 MILLION PEOPLE ARE TAKING AT LEAST one herbal remedy or natural supplement, along with their prescription medications. Studies demonstrate that people may not tell their physicians or health-care providers about their supplements. However, it's important to note that your health-care provider needs to know which natural remedies you are taking because of the risk of drug-supplement interactions.

In this chapter, my goal is to give you a working knowledge of the common supplements I see people taking or asking about on a routine basis. The benefits and risks of natural products are not as well understood because many of the studies assessing their efficacy are limited. Also, in many cases, the clinical data is anecdotal. That said, both medications and natural supplements are versatile and can have applications for many health conditions. For example, ACE inhibitors are not just medications prescribed for the treatment of high blood pressure; they also have heart- and kidney-protective effects and improve the mortality rate in individuals with chronic heart failure. Likewise, natural supplements can be used for a variety of health conditions. Turmeric, for example, has been cited by articles as an effective supplement in the treatment of pain, cardiovascular health, and liver health. Magnesium also has many uses, including the treatment of pain, high blood pressure, and perhaps even diabetes.

While the list of supplements in this chapter is not exhaustive, many practical uses and concerns regarding supplements are discussed. Supplements are organized in this chapter based on the condition for which they are most commonly and beneficially used.

Not all supplements are created alike. You should make sure that the supplement you are using is pure and contains active ingredients. Some companies that make natural supplements do so following standards set by the U.S. Pharmacopeial Convention. Generally, those are the most reliable. Look for a USP label or a label that states that the products have been independently verified for active ingredients by an outside lab. A GMP (good manufacturing practice) seal is not sufficient because it only verifies that the manufacturing is done well—not that the supplement contains active ingredients. Do not hesitate to contact a health professional or a pharmacist if you have questions concerning a particular supplement or brand.

Neither medications nor natural supplements are a substitute for a healthy diet and daily exercise plan, and they should not be an excuse to eat unhealthily. With that in mind, I believe that natural supplements can be integrated successfully into a personalized treatment plan for many health conditions.

As echoed throughout this book, if you have any questions concerning the use of natural supplements, do not hesitate to ask your doctor or pharmacist. In addition, there are helpful online guides, some of which are listed in the Resources section.

* * *

Do You Really Need to Take Supplements?

This is one of the common questions asked by many people who are taking several medications. I answer, "It depends," to this question for a couple reasons:

- If your daily food consumption consists primarily of processed foods and fast foods, you likely have significant nutrient deficiencies that need to be addressed. These deficiencies can contribute to chronic illness. On the other hand, if you are eating a healthy diet that is nutrient-dense and includes plenty of fruits and vegetables, it is less likely that you need additional supplementation.
- If you are taking prescription medications, you likely have nutrient deficiencies induced by them. For example, thiazide diuretics prescribed for the treatment of high blood pressure can lead to very low potassium and magnesium levels.

* * *

Pain Relief Supplements

One of the biggest struggles that health-care providers have is treating pain, especially chronic pain. The risks associated with narcotic pain medications and NSAIDs that you read about in chapter 8 can sometimes outweigh the benefits. A combination of supplements can be used together, or synergistically, for maximal pain relief in those patients who may not tolerate certain prescription painkillers.

1 Which (if any) of the following supplements are you taking for pain relief?

☐ Alpha lipoic acid

☐ Arnica montana

☐ Boswellia extract

☐ Devil's claw

☐ Topical magnesium

☐ Omega-3 fish oil

☐ Probiotics

☐ Tart cherry extract

☐ Turmeric

☐ Wobenzym® N

☐ Other: _____

- Above are some of the common supplements that people take for pain relief. Many people, in fact, take more than one supplement for this purpose. If you are doing so, it is important to discuss them with your doctor. When too many pills and supplements are taken, it can be difficult to ascertain which supplement or medication may be producing side effects, if they develop.

2 What is the cause of your pain?

☐ Arthritis, including osteoarthritis or gout

☐ Neuropathy, including diabetic neuropathy

☐ Muscle injury or strain

☐ Other: _____

☐ I don't know.

- Alpha lipoic acid can be of tremendous help for nerve pain (including diabetic neuropathy), although it can take several weeks to take effect. There are many studies demonstrating its successful use, along with prescription medication, for the treatment of neuropathy.

- Arnica montana is a homeopathic remedy that can help with the treatment of arthritis. Two impressive studies showed that Arnica montana can reduce pain and improve functioning in individuals suffering from osteoarthritis of the hands and knees.

- The topical form of magnesium can help relieve pain in muscles and joints if you have severe arthritis. In fact, some athletes use this for pain relief after strenuous workouts.

- In addition to treating high triglyceride levels, omega-3 fish oil has been shown to have anti-inflammatory properties.

- Probiotics help to reduce inflammation systemically, and if you can reduce inflammation, you can reduce pain. The usage of probiotics is highlighted later in this chapter.

- Tart cherry extract is excellent for arthritis and also has been shown in studies to help athletes reduce pain after exercise.

- Turmeric is terrific for pain relief. It is a potent anti-inflammatory agent, and in one study 1,500 mg daily was shown to be as effective as 1,200 mg of ibuprofen in reducing knee pain over a four-week period.

....

THE PERSONALIZED APPROACH
Treating Arthritis with Natural Agents

The following example shows how replacing prescription painkillers with a mix of pain-relief supplements can create a successful personalized pain-treatment plan for patients with suboptimal kidney and/or liver function:

Mr. L is a gentleman in his sixties who has been suffering from significant knee arthritis. He has not been able to tolerate prescription medications due to side effects, and given that his kidney function is compromised, he has not been able to take over-the-counter NSAIDs, such as Advil or Aleve. On his last office visit, four months prior, he was prescribed topical Arnica montana. He applied it to his knees twice daily from then on and noticed a significant decrease in his pain levels. He recorded his physical activity with a pedometer and found that, despite walking more than 16,000 steps a day, his pain was dramatically reduced. As you will read, Arnica montana is a homeopathic medication with anti-inflammatory properties and minimal side effects.

My goal in treating Mr. L with anti-inflammatory supplements is to decrease the frequency and duration of NSAID and/or narcotic painkillers and improve his quality of life. While replacing potent medications with natural agents is not a foolproof solution, it allows doctors to reduce the number of prescription medications someone is taking and the associated risk of their side effects.

....

3 What dose are you currently taking, at what frequency?
———— mg ———— times a day.

- I recommend beginning with a low dose (100–200 mg daily) of alpha lipoic acid, which can be increased slowly up to 300–600 mg in divided doses. This supplement can be taken twice a day.

- Arnica montana can be taken sublingually (under the tongue) or topically—i.e., directly applied to the area of inflammation. I recommend rubbing the Arnica montana 30× dosage on the affected area twice a day if. If you prefer the sublingual form, this can be taken two to three times a day. If you have diffuse arthritis, I advise trying both forms together.

- Common dosing regimens for fish oil start at 2 g a day and can be increased to 3–4 g a day.

- Magnesium is not just something that you can take orally. Believe it or not, it also comes as a gel and an oil that can be topically applied twice a day. Athletes rub it on sore areas after a workout, for example. (Caution: Some people may develop a contact allergy to topical magnesium.)

- Take one ounce of tart cherry extract twice a day to start. (Tip: Many people will take this in a shot glass. If you have diabetes, this should not raise your blood glucose levels.)

- I recommend starting turmeric at 500 mg daily and then increasing to twice a day. Most people take between one and two grams a day.

- Although Wobenzym N can help to relieve inflammation and pain, you may end up taking six to twelve tablets a day before you notice some improvement in pain and inflammation.

* * *

SUPPLEMENT SPOTLIGHT

Probiotics

There are many different types and classes of probiotics, so this question often comes up: What should I be looking for in a probiotic?

There are trillions of bacteria in your GI tract. Many probiotics provide 3 to 5 million colony-forming units (CFU) of bacteria per capsule. Look at the ingredients of your probiotic—they should contain species of *Lactobacillus* and *Bifidobacterium* at minimum.

One of the main side effects of probiotics is diarrhea and loose stools. There might be an increase in the frequency of bowel movements, which can be intolerable for some people. However, it is important to understand that a person should have one to two bowel movements daily for optimal health.

If you are taking an antibiotic, you should take a probiotic as well to help preserve the health of your intestine. However, it should be taken at a different time of the day. There are many studies looking at other health benefits of probiotics, including inflammation reduction, lowering of cholesterol, and blood pressure reduction. Some studies even suggest a benefit to the immune system and infections of the respiratory system. There can be many potential benefits of taking probiotics!

* * *

4. Have you been diagnosed with any of the following conditions?

☐ Diabetes

☐ DVT or a blood-clotting disorder

☐ Atrial fibrillation

- Because alpha lipoic acid can decrease insulin resistance, which leads to lower blood glucose levels, you need to follow your blood glucose levels closely if you have diabetes.

- If you are on blood thinners because of DVT, atrial fibrillation, or some other reason, be mindful that omega-3 fish oil can also thin the blood.

* * *

CONDITION SPOTLIGHT

Gout

....

Gout is an extremely painful arthritic condition that is caused by the deposition of uric acid crystals into the joints. It commonly affects older males. The most frequent initial symptom is pain in the big toe, but pain can also start in the knee, shoulder, or wrist. It sometimes occurs in multiple joints. If you have ever suffered a "gout flare," you can testify to how painful and debilitating it can be.

Common prescription medications for the treatment of acute gout include colchicine (Colcrys®), while allopurinol (Zyloprim) and febuxostat (Uloric) are popular treatments for chronic gout. In addition to interfering with the production of uric acid, febuxostat may also decrease the amount of tophi (uric acid crystal deposits) in the joints.

Yet, there are supplements that you can use in addition to medications for the treatment of a painful gout flare. In one study, the use of allopurinol in combination with tart cherry extract helped to decrease the duration and severity of the gout flare by 75 percent. I tend to recommend an average dose of 1–2 oz daily to my gout patients. Believe it or not, the use of probiotics can decrease uric acid levels. Be sure you are taking them at least once a day as part of your daily supplement regimen if you have been diagnosed with gout.

* * *

Energy Supplements

Fatigue and loss of energy are among the common reasons that people visit their doctors. We can't stress enough the importance of communicating with your doctor about fatigue that is chronic or severe, as your doctor may need to evaluate blood counts to be sure that you are not anemic, your kidney and liver functions are in good working order, and you don't have an underactive thyroid, or hypothyroidism. *Note that the supplements discussed in this section are cited by some as improving energy at the level of the cell; we are not talking about substances that have "brain stimulant" properties.*

1 Which (if any) of the following supplements are you taking to boost your energy level?

☐ Ubiquinone (coenzyme Q_{10})

☐ Magnesium

☐ D-ribose

☐ Vitamin C

☐ Vitamin B complex

☐ Other: _____

- Ubiquinone (coenzyme Q_{10}) is a substance located in cell mitochondria that aids in the process of generating energy. Some recent studies suggest that mitochondrial dysfunction and coenzyme Q_{10} deficiency may be to blame for symptoms of fibromyalgia and certain other chronic illnesses, so many holistic health practitioners prescribe coenzyme Q_{10} to restore mitochondrial function and increase mitochondrial biogenesis, which has been linked to improved muscle strength and a reduction in muscle pain and fatigue.

- The adrenal gland needs vitamin C and vitamin B complex for optimal functioning.

SUPPLEMENT SPOTLIGHT

Magnesium

....

Magnesium does so many things! It helps with pain, it can help improve energy, and it also can help you sleep if you take it at night before you go to bed. Magnesium supplementation can also help to regulate your blood pressure as well as treat migraines. A divided oral dose of 400–600 mg is usually taken throughout the day, with at least one dose taken before bedtime.

Tip: In some people, magnesium supplementation can cause diarrhea, so if you notice this effect, you should look for another form of magnesium. The lactate and acetate forms of magnesium cause less diarrhea, as compared with the other magnesium formulations. One other option is to take magnesium with calcium (which is more constipating and can cancel out the effect of magnesium).

* * *

2 What is the cause of your fatigue?

☐ Chronic illness

☐ Fibromyalgia

☐ Insomnia

☐ Other: _____

☐ I don't know.

- Fatigue can result from chronic illness and fibromyalgia, which can also cause significant pain and weakness. Many people with fibromyalgia are unable to get a good night's sleep because of the pain, which obviously affects their energy level. As such, part of the treatment strategy for improving energy also involves taking supplements, such as melatonin, that help you get a good night's sleep. See chapter 5 for more information on this supplement.

3 What dose are you currently taking, at what frequency?

_____ mg _____ times a day.

- Ubiquinone (coenzyme Q_{10}) can be taken at doses of 50–100 mg, daily to start and increased to be taken at least twice a day.

- While it does come in capsule form, I recommend the powdered form of D-ribose. A good starting dose is 2,500 mg, which can be increased to 5,000 mg. Recalling Mr. N's testimony in the introduction (see page v), this patient found that 5,000 mg of D-ribose dramatically improved his energy level.

- Patients seeking increased energy should take at least 2,000 mg of vitamin C daily, along with a good B complex vitamin. The ester form of vitamin C is thought to be better absorbed.

4 Have you experienced any of the following symptoms while taking this supplement?

☐ Diarrhea

☐ Stomach upset or heartburn

☐ Dizziness or lightheadedness

☐ Other: _____

- Too high of a dose of D-ribose can cause diarrhea.

- Some patients have reported stomach upset or mild heartburn when taking ubiquinone (coenzyme Q_{10}), which stopped when the dose was decreased or taken with food.

- In some individuals, ubiquinone (coenzyme Q_{10}) may decrease blood pressure, so if you are taking this supplement along with other blood pressure medications, monitor your blood pressure.

* * *

SUPPLEMENT SPOTLIGHT

Vitamin D

Our nation is one of extensive vitamin D deficiency, so you should consider asking your doctor to have your vitamin D levels measured. Low vitamin D levels can affect a lot of things, including illness susceptibility, anemia, heart function, diabetes risk, bone health, and even your energy level. One key role of vitamin D in the body, besides its critical function in helping the body absorb calcium for strong bones, is aiding the conversion of tryptophan into serotonin, and some studies suggest it has an antidepressant effect.

If it is necessary to supplement vitamin D, your dosage will depend on how low your blood level is as well as your body build. Doses of vitamin D_3 can range from 1,000 to 5,000 international units (IU) daily, or 50,000 IU of vitamin D_2 may be recommended to be taken once a week.

* * *

Cholesterol-Lowering Supplements

Some natural supplements can be used to lower blood triglycerides and "optimize" your cholesterol profile to improve your heart health. Conveniently, many of these natural agents can be taken at the same time that you take your prescription medications.

1 Which (if any) of the following supplements are you currently taking to reduce cholesterol?

☐ Red yeast rice

☐ Omega-3 fish oil

☐ Plant phytosterols

☐ Fiber

☐ Other: _____

- Red yeast rice is probably the most common supplement that we see patients taking to help reduce cholesterol. Note, however, that a significant chemical component of red yeast rice is identical to lovastatin, so you should never take it with other statin medications.

- Omega-3 fish oil is effective for reducing triglyceride levels.

- Plant phytosterols such as beta-sitosterol can be used to help reduce total cholesterol levels. If you are a man, beta-sitosterol has an added benefit: it can help in the treatment of an enlarged prostate (BPH).

- Fiber—found in many foods, particularly vegetables, legumes, and fruits—helps to reduce serum cholesterol. Soluble fiber can be obtained in supplements like Metamucil® and Citrucel®, which are mixed into water. (Foods such as oats, barley, and legumes contain soluble fiber, in addition to the products mentioned above.)

2 What dose are you currently taking, at what frequency?

_____ mg _____ times a day.

- I usually suggest starting on 600 mg a day of red yeast rice and slowly increasing the dose over a period of weeks. A usual maximum dose is 1,200 mg, taken twice a day. *Please do not consume red yeast rice if you are taking a statin, fibrate, or niacin medication. One or the other may be taken to reduce cholesterol, but not both.*

- I usually prescribe a starting dose of at least 1,000 mg a day of omega-3 fish oil.

- If you are taking a fiber supplement such as Metamucil in the morning, be sure that you mix a heaping tablespoonful of fiber in at least six to eight ounces of water for maximum absorption.

3 Have you experienced any of the following symptoms while taking this supplement?

- ☐ Unexplained pain in your muscles or joints

- ☐ Difficulty walking because of pain or fatigue

- ☐ Blood in the urine

- ☐ Signs of liver or kidney damage, including yellowing of the eyes or skin, increased fatigue, decreased urine output, or tea-colored urine

- ☐ Other: _____

- While it is "natural," you need to let your doctor know if you are taking red yeast rice because it can cause many of the same side effects as statins, including increased liver enzymes and myopathy. *Stop taking this supplement if you experience these side effects.* You will need to have your liver function monitored as well.

4 Are you taking any of the following medications that might interact with this supplement?

- ☐ Statins

- ☐ Fibrates

- ☐ Niacin

- As suggested above, do not take red yeast rice with other statins, fibrates, or niacin, as the combination can increase the risk of developing liver and kidney problems.

- Plant sterols, on the other hand, can be taken safely with other statins and fibrates to reduce cholesterol levels.

* * *

CONDITION SPOTLIGHT

Recurrent UTIs

If you have taken multiple rounds of antibiotics for the treatment of recurrent urinary tract infections (UTIs), believe it or not, supplements can help. Maintaining a healthy bowel flora can be of tremendous help in reducing recurrent

UTIs, so taking a probiotic may be a good idea. Also, certain types of bacteria that frequently cause UTIs, such as *E. coli*, stick to the lining of your urinary tract in much the same way that Spiderman sticks to walls. Luckily, the use of cranberry extract can help decrease the "stickiness" of the *E. coli* in the urinary tract. I often recommend that those with frequent UTIs consider taking the powder form of D-mannose, 500–1,000 mg a day, to treat existing UTIs as well as prevent their recurrence.

* * *

Supplements for Diabetes

Many people are looking for natural supplements to help reduce blood glucose levels. Some of the supplements included in this section can also help in the treatment of metabolic syndrome, which raises your risk of diabetes and heart disease.

1 Which (if any) of the following supplements are you taking for diabetes?

- ☐ Chromium picolinate
- ☐ Alpha lipoic acid
- ☐ Fiber
- ☐ Turmeric
- ☐ Probiotics
- ☐ Fenugreek
- ☐ Gymnema sylvestre
- ☐ Ubiquinone (coenzyme Q_{10})
- ☐ Magnesium
- ☐ Other: _____

- Chromium picolinate and alpha lipoic acid can help decrease insulin resistance by helping insulin to enter the cells.

- Fiber can slow down the absorption of carbohydrates and glucose in the body by binding to them.

- Probiotics, by helping to normalize intestinal flora, can help to normalize blood glucose levels.

- Fenugreek is an herb that has been demonstrated to help decrease blood glucose levels.

- Some of the prescription diabetes medications, including the oral sulfonylureas, can deplete the body of ubiquinone (coenzyme Q_{10}), so it should be supplemented.

- Magnesium has been shown in some studies to help improve insulin resistance.

2 What dose are you currently taking, at what frequency?

_____ mg _____ times a day.

- I recommend 100–200 micrograms of chromium picolinate a day.

- Ubiquinone (coenzyme Q_{10}) supplementation usually starts at 50–100 mg a day.

- Standard dosage of magnesium is 400–600 mg a day.

3 Have you experienced any of the following symptoms while taking this supplement?

☐ Symptoms of hypoglycemia (dizziness, sweating, increased irritability, and confusion)

- If you are taking any supplements for diabetes, it is important that you speak with your doctor about them. Because of the risk of hypoglycemia, you may need to decrease the dosage of your prescription diabetes medications or even discontinue them completely. You should do so under the guidance of a physician or health-care professional.

4 Are you taking any of the following medications that might interact with this supplement?

☐ Quinolone antibiotics

☐ Diabetes medications

☐ Blood thinners

- Quinolones and diabetes medications can cause low blood glucose levels, so it is important to monitor your blood glucose levels closely if you are taking these medications in addition to your diabetes supplement.

- If you are taking any blood thinners, speak with your doctor before taking turmeric, as it can further thin the blood.

Fiber for Gastrointestinal Health

Because gastrointestinal health is one of the most common reasons that people see a health-care professional, many are taking over-the-counter supplements and herbs to help their symptoms. Some of the most popular and effective supplements intended for this purpose include probiotics, digestive enzymes, and fiber.

Probiotics are live bacteria that help to promote gut health. (For details about these useful supplements, see page 168.) Digestive enzymes are also recommended by many holistic health practitioners to help the GI tract to break down and absorb nutrients. Additionally, fiber is key to gut health, helping to regulate bowel movements.

It is recommended that everyone get at least 20–25 grams of fiber daily for optimum GI health. Most of us do not have enough fiber in our diet, so in many cases it needs to be supplemented by other means. Available in many forms, fiber consists of two types: soluble and insoluble. Soluble fiber absorbs water in your food, slowing digestion, while insoluble fiber adds bulk to stools, easing constipation. The most common fiber supplements are psyllium-based, containing 70 percent soluble fiber and 30 percent insoluble fiber. Metamucil, for example, is psyllium sold in capsule or powder form. I tend to recommend one heaping tablespoon of psyllium powder in an eight-ounce glass of water for optimum results.

Some people may develop significant flatulence and possibly stomach upset when taking certain types of fiber supplements, but in those situations, they can work with their doctors to find acceptable alternatives. Note that fiber may affect the absorption of other medications and should be taken separately. For example, if you need to take your medications early in the morning, take your fiber around lunchtime.

Fiber has a lot of important functions besides maintaining a healthy gut. There is evidence that fiber has heart- and liver-protective effects. It can also help control blood sugar levels in diabetic and pre-diabetic individuals and lower blood pressure. Daily fiber intake is also associated with weight loss, and insoluble fiber may decrease your risk of colon cancer.

* * *

Blood Pressure–Lowering Supplements

There are many valuable supplements that can help improve heart health and blood pressure. Many people will take more than one supplement for this purpose, and it is the combination that can have beneficial effects.

1 Which (if any) of the following supplements are you currently taking to lower blood pressure?

- ☐ Magnesium
- ☐ Ubiquinone (coenzyme Q_{10})
- ☐ Garlic
- ☐ Turmeric
- ☐ Dark chocolate
- ☐ Olive leaf extract
- ☐ Other: _____

- Low magnesium consumption can increase the risk of developing high blood pressure and stroke. In addition to magnesium supplementation, increasing your consumption of green leafy vegetables, nuts, and seeds—all of which have high magnesium content—is helpful, too.

- Ubiquinone (coenzyme Q_{10}) helps to stabilize the inner lining of the blood vessel called the endothelium. The dysfunction of this lining is thought to contribute to the development of hypertension.

- The use of aged garlic extract can also help lower blood pressure, since garlic is an effective "dilator" of blood vessels.

- Turmeric has excellent natural anti-inflammatory and antioxidant properties. Inflammation is implicated in numerous conditions, including high blood pressure and heart disease.

- There has been a lot of recent data concerning dark chocolate and its blood pressure–lowering effect, as cocoa is high in antioxidants. The key with dark chocolate is that it needs to have minimal sugar content.

- Olive leaf extract does have blood pressure–lowering effects, as well as other exceptional antioxidant properties.

2 What dose are you currently taking, at what frequency?

_____ mg _____ times a day.

- While there are a variety of magnesium supplements available, my personal preference is to take the chelated form in doses of 200–400 mg on a daily basis.

- Ubiquinone (coenzyme Q_{10}) can be started at doses of 50–100 mg once a day, eventually increasing to twice a day.

- The degree to which garlic can decrease blood pressure seems to be dose dependent. Start at 200–300 mg daily and increase the dosage slowly.

- Turmeric can be started at 500 mg to 1 g and increased slowly.

- In one study cited, the dose of olive leaf extract needed to sustain a blood pressure–lowering effect was 500 mg, twice a day.

3 Have you experienced any of the following symptoms while taking this supplement?

☐ Dizziness or lightheadedness, especially upon standing

☐ Stomach upset

☐ Nausea

☐ Diarrhea

☐ Other: _____

- Be aware that any supplement that lowers blood pressure, especially when taken in conjunction with blood pressure medications, may cause dizziness and lightheadedness.

- Some blood pressure–lowering supplements may cause mild stomach upset and/or nausea within the first few days of starting them. These symptoms should dissipate after a few days, but if you find that they persist, stop the supplement and speak with your doctor.

- As mentioned on page 171, magnesium can cause diarrhea in some individuals. Taking a constipating supplement such as calcium may cancel out this side effect.

4 Are you taking any of the following medications that might interact with this supplement?

☐ Blood thinners

☐ Blood pressure medications

- Garlic and turmeric have blood-thinning properties, so their dosages should be monitored and possibly reduced if you are taking other blood thinners.

- As mentioned previously, supplements that lower blood pressure combined with blood pressure–lowering prescription medications may make your blood pressure too low.

* * *

DOCTOR'S SPOTLIGHT

Is There a Role for Preventive Supplementation?

Frequently, patients ask me if they should be taking supplements preventively, even if they have no specific medical problem. In fact, the right supplements— in combination with a proper diet and exercise plan—can help keep us healthy and prevent or delay the onset of the chronic illnesses that dominate our modern medical landscape. Here is a list of the supplements that I take "preventively" and often recommend to patients:

- *Coenzyme Q$_{10}$* for heart and cellular health, as well as an energy boost.
- *Magnesium* for heart and brain health, as well as diabetes prevention.
- *Turmeric* for liver health, heart health, brain health, kidney health, pain and inflammation reduction, and cancer prevention.
- *Vitamin D* for heart health, bone health, and inflammation reduction.
- *Probiotics* for a healthy immune system and GI tract, as well as inflammation reduction.
- A *multivitamin* for optimal levels of important vitamins and nutrients and to prevent deficiencies.

Note that some practitioners can do specialized testing to identify key nutrient deficiencies beyond those identified in standard blood tests. They can also help to personalize your nutrient plan. Further discussion on this is beyond the scope of this book, but the "big six" mentioned above are good options for most people in industrialized countries. If nothing else, it is a starting point for better health.

* * *

Notes

Notes

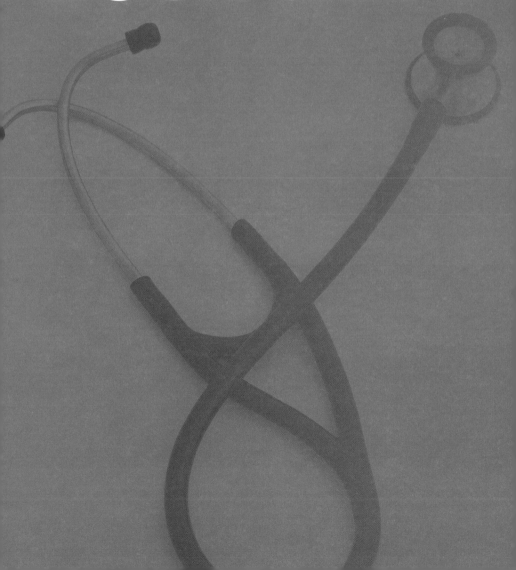

Doctor Visits & Test Results

Doctor Visits & Test Results

APPOINTMENT DATE _6 / 15 / 16_   TIME _1:30 PM_
DOCTOR _DR. FOWLER_   SPECIALTY _NEPHROLOGY_
LOCATION _CEDARS-SINAI_   PHONE _____

PURPOSE OF VISIT:
_____
_____
_____

SYMPTOMS & CONCERNS:
LOWER BACK PAIN, BLOOD IN URINE—POSSIBLE KIDNEY STONE?
_____

VITAL SIGNS AND STATS
☑ HEIGHT _5' 8"_   ☑ HEART RATE _98_
☑ WEIGHT _143 LBS_   ☐ WAIST CIRCUMFERENCE _____
☑ BLOOD PRESSURE _130 / 80_   ☑ TEMPERATURE _99.7_

TESTS ORDERED
☑ URINALYSIS   ☐ X-RAY/CT SCAN
☑ CBC BLOOD TEST   ☑ ULTRASOUND
☐ BASIC METABOLIC PANEL (CHEM)   ☑ OTHER _UREA NITROGEN_
☐ LIVER FUNCTION TEST   ☑ OTHER _CREATININE_
☐ THYROID FUNCTION TESTS   ☐ OTHER _____

DOCTOR INSTRUCTIONS:
DRINK LOTS OF WATER, IBUPROFEN FOR PAIN
_____
_____

ABNORMAL RESULTS:
ELEVATED UN, CREATININE
_____
_____

OTHER NOTES:
No KIDNEY STONE DETECTED. ANTIBIOTIC FOR KIDNEY INFECTION
TO BE TAKEN 2x PER DAY.
_____

SAMPLE

APPOINTMENT DATE _____   TIME _____

DOCTOR _____   SPECIALTY _____

LOCATION _____   PHONE _____

PURPOSE OF VISIT: _____

_____

_____

SYMPTOMS & CONCERNS: _____

_____

_____

VITAL SIGNS AND STATS

☐ HEIGHT _____   ☐ HEART RATE _____

☐ WEIGHT _____   ☐ WAIST CIRCUMFERENCE _____

☐ BLOOD PRESSURE _____   ☐ TEMPERATURE _____

TESTS ORDERED

☐ URINALYSIS   ☐ X-RAY/CT SCAN

☐ CBC BLOOD TEST   ☐ ULTRASOUND

☐ BASIC METABOLIC PANEL (CHEM)   ☐ OTHER _____

☐ LIVER FUNCTION TEST   ☐ OTHER _____

☐ THYROID FUNCTION TESTS   ☐ OTHER _____

DOCTOR INSTRUCTIONS: _____

_____

_____

_____

ABNORMAL RESULTS: _____

_____

_____

_____

OTHER NOTES: _____

_____

_____

_____

APPOINTMENT DATE _____ TIME _____

DOCTOR _____ SPECIALTY _____

LOCATION _____ PHONE _____

PURPOSE OF VISIT: _____
_____
_____

SYMPTOMS & CONCERNS: _____
_____
_____

VITAL SIGNS AND STATS

- [ ] HEIGHT _____
- [ ] WEIGHT _____
- [ ] BLOOD PRESSURE _____

- [ ] HEART RATE _____
- [ ] WAIST CIRCUMFERENCE _____
- [ ] TEMPERATURE _____

TESTS ORDERED

- [ ] URINALYSIS
- [ ] CBC BLOOD TEST
- [ ] BASIC METABOLIC PANEL (CHEM)
- [ ] LIVER FUNCTION TEST
- [ ] THYROID FUNCTION TESTS

- [ ] X-RAY/CT SCAN
- [ ] ULTRASOUND
- [ ] OTHER _____
- [ ] OTHER _____
- [ ] OTHER _____

DOCTOR INSTRUCTIONS: _____
_____
_____
_____

ABNORMAL RESULTS: _____
_____
_____
_____

OTHER NOTES: _____
_____
_____
_____

APPOINTMENT DATE _____   TIME _____

DOCTOR _____   SPECIALTY _____

LOCATION _____   PHONE _____

PURPOSE OF VISIT: _____

_____

_____

SYMPTOMS & CONCERNS: _____

_____

_____

VITAL SIGNS AND STATS

☐ HEIGHT _____   ☐ HEART RATE _____

☐ WEIGHT _____   ☐ WAIST CIRCUMFERENCE _____

☐ BLOOD PRESSURE _____   ☐ TEMPERATURE _____

TESTS ORDERED

☐ URINALYSIS   ☐ X-RAY/CT SCAN

☐ CBC BLOOD TEST   ☐ ULTRASOUND

☐ BASIC METABOLIC PANEL (CHEM)   ☐ OTHER _____

☐ LIVER FUNCTION TEST   ☐ OTHER _____

☐ THYROID FUNCTION TESTS   ☐ OTHER _____

DOCTOR INSTRUCTIONS: _____

_____

_____

_____

ABNORMAL RESULTS: _____

_____

_____

_____

OTHER NOTES: _____

_____

_____

_____

APPOINTMENT DATE _____   TIME _____

DOCTOR _____   SPECIALTY _____

LOCATION _____   PHONE _____

PURPOSE OF VISIT: _____

_____

_____

SYMPTOMS & CONCERNS: _____

_____

_____

VITAL SIGNS AND STATS

☐ HEIGHT _____   ☐ HEART RATE _____

☐ WEIGHT _____   ☐ WAIST CIRCUMFERENCE _____

☐ BLOOD PRESSURE _____   ☐ TEMPERATURE _____

TESTS ORDERED

☐ URINALYSIS   ☐ X-RAY/CT SCAN

☐ CBC BLOOD TEST   ☐ ULTRASOUND

☐ BASIC METABOLIC PANEL (CHEM)   ☐ OTHER _____

☐ LIVER FUNCTION TEST   ☐ OTHER _____

☐ THYROID FUNCTION TESTS   ☐ OTHER _____

DOCTOR INSTRUCTIONS: _____

_____

_____

_____

ABNORMAL RESULTS: _____

_____

_____

_____

OTHER NOTES: _____

_____

_____

_____

APPOINTMENT DATE _____   TIME _____

DOCTOR _____   SPECIALTY _____

LOCATION _____   PHONE _____

PURPOSE OF VISIT: _____

_____

_____

SYMPTOMS & CONCERNS: _____

_____

_____

VITAL SIGNS AND STATS

☐ HEIGHT _____   ☐ HEART RATE _____

☐ WEIGHT _____   ☐ WAIST CIRCUMFERENCE _____

☐ BLOOD PRESSURE _____   ☐ TEMPERATURE _____

TESTS ORDERED

☐ URINALYSIS   ☐ X-RAY/CT SCAN

☐ CBC BLOOD TEST   ☐ ULTRASOUND

☐ BASIC METABOLIC PANEL (CHEM)   ☐ OTHER _____

☐ LIVER FUNCTION TEST   ☐ OTHER _____

☐ THYROID FUNCTION TESTS   ☐ OTHER _____

DOCTOR INSTRUCTIONS: _____

_____

_____

_____

ABNORMAL RESULTS: _____

_____

_____

_____

OTHER NOTES: _____

_____

_____

_____

APPOINTMENT DATE ——————— TIME ———————————

DOCTOR ——————————— SPECIALTY ———————————

LOCATION ——————————— PHONE ———————————

PURPOSE OF VISIT: ———————————————————

———————————————————————

———————————————————————

SYMPTOMS & CONCERNS: ———————————————

———————————————————————

———————————————————————

VITAL SIGNS AND STATS

☐ HEIGHT ————————— ☐ HEART RATE ——————

☐ WEIGHT ————————— ☐ WAIST CIRCUMFERENCE ————

☐ BLOOD PRESSURE ————— ☐ TEMPERATURE —————

TESTS ORDERED

☐ URINALYSIS ☐ X-RAY/CT SCAN

☐ CBC BLOOD TEST ☐ ULTRASOUND

☐ BASIC METABOLIC PANEL (CHEM) ☐ OTHER ——————

☐ LIVER FUNCTION TEST ☐ OTHER ——————

☐ THYROID FUNCTION TESTS ☐ OTHER ——————

DOCTOR INSTRUCTIONS: ———————————————

———————————————————————

———————————————————————

———————————————————————

ABNORMAL RESULTS: —————————————————

———————————————————————

———————————————————————

———————————————————————

OTHER NOTES: ————————————————————

———————————————————————

———————————————————————

———————————————————————

APPOINTMENT DATE _____   TIME _____

DOCTOR _____   SPECIALTY _____

LOCATION _____   PHONE _____

PURPOSE OF VISIT: _____

_____

_____

SYMPTOMS & CONCERNS: _____

_____

_____

VITAL SIGNS AND STATS

☐ HEIGHT _____   ☐ HEART RATE _____

☐ WEIGHT _____   ☐ WAIST CIRCUMFERENCE _____

☐ BLOOD PRESSURE _____   ☐ TEMPERATURE _____

TESTS ORDERED

☐ URINALYSIS   ☐ X-RAY/CT SCAN

☐ CBC BLOOD TEST   ☐ ULTRASOUND

☐ BASIC METABOLIC PANEL (CHEM)   ☐ OTHER _____

☐ LIVER FUNCTION TEST   ☐ OTHER _____

☐ THYROID FUNCTION TESTS   ☐ OTHER _____

DOCTOR INSTRUCTIONS: _____

_____

_____

_____

ABNORMAL RESULTS: _____

_____

_____

_____

OTHER NOTES: _____

_____

_____

_____

APPOINTMENT DATE _____   TIME _____

DOCTOR _____   SPECIALTY _____

LOCATION _____   PHONE _____

PURPOSE OF VISIT: _____

_____

_____

SYMPTOMS & CONCERNS: _____

_____

_____

VITAL SIGNS AND STATS

☐ HEIGHT _____   ☐ HEART RATE _____

☐ WEIGHT _____   ☐ WAIST CIRCUMFERENCE _____

☐ BLOOD PRESSURE _____   ☐ TEMPERATURE _____

TESTS ORDERED

☐ URINALYSIS   ☐ X-RAY/CT SCAN

☐ CBC BLOOD TEST   ☐ ULTRASOUND

☐ BASIC METABOLIC PANEL (CHEM)   ☐ OTHER _____

☐ LIVER FUNCTION TEST   ☐ OTHER _____

☐ THYROID FUNCTION TESTS   ☐ OTHER _____

DOCTOR INSTRUCTIONS: _____

_____

_____

_____

ABNORMAL RESULTS: _____

_____

_____

_____

OTHER NOTES: _____

_____

_____

_____

APPOINTMENT DATE _____   TIME _____

DOCTOR _____   SPECIALTY _____

LOCATION _____   PHONE _____

PURPOSE OF VISIT: _____

_____

_____

SYMPTOMS & CONCERNS: _____

_____

_____

VITAL SIGNS AND STATS

☐ HEIGHT _____   ☐ HEART RATE _____

☐ WEIGHT _____   ☐ WAIST CIRCUMFERENCE _____

☐ BLOOD PRESSURE _____ ☐ TEMPERATURE _____

TESTS ORDERED

☐ URINALYSIS   ☐ X-RAY/CT SCAN

☐ CBC BLOOD TEST   ☐ ULTRASOUND

☐ BASIC METABOLIC PANEL (CHEM)   ☐ OTHER _____

☐ LIVER FUNCTION TEST   ☐ OTHER _____

☐ THYROID FUNCTION TESTS   ☐ OTHER _____

DOCTOR INSTRUCTIONS: _____

_____

_____

_____

ABNORMAL RESULTS: _____

_____

_____

_____

OTHER NOTES: _____

_____

_____

_____

APPOINTMENT DATE _____   TIME _____
DOCTOR _____   SPECIALTY _____
LOCATION _____   PHONE _____

PURPOSE OF VISIT: _____
_____
_____
_____

SYMPTOMS & CONCERNS: _____
_____
_____
_____

VITAL SIGNS AND STATS
☐ HEIGHT _____   ☐ HEART RATE _____
☐ WEIGHT _____   ☐ WAIST CIRCUMFERENCE _____
☐ BLOOD PRESSURE _____   ☐ TEMPERATURE _____

TESTS ORDERED
☐ URINALYSIS   ☐ X-RAY/CT SCAN
☐ CBC BLOOD TEST   ☐ ULTRASOUND
☐ BASIC METABOLIC PANEL (CHEM)   ☐ OTHER _____
☐ LIVER FUNCTION TEST   ☐ OTHER _____
☐ THYROID FUNCTION TESTS   ☐ OTHER _____

DOCTOR INSTRUCTIONS: _____
_____
_____
_____
_____

ABNORMAL RESULTS: _____
_____
_____
_____
_____

OTHER NOTES: _____
_____
_____
_____
_____

APPOINTMENT DATE _____   TIME _____

DOCTOR _____   SPECIALTY _____

LOCATION _____   PHONE _____

PURPOSE OF VISIT: _____

_____

_____

SYMPTOMS & CONCERNS: _____

_____

_____

VITAL SIGNS AND STATS

☐ HEIGHT _____   ☐ HEART RATE _____

☐ WEIGHT _____   ☐ WAIST CIRCUMFERENCE _____

☐ BLOOD PRESSURE _____   ☐ TEMPERATURE _____

TESTS ORDERED

☐ URINALYSIS   ☐ X-RAY/CT SCAN

☐ CBC BLOOD TEST   ☐ ULTRASOUND

☐ BASIC METABOLIC PANEL (CHEM)   ☐ OTHER _____

☐ LIVER FUNCTION TEST   ☐ OTHER _____

☐ THYROID FUNCTION TESTS   ☐ OTHER _____

DOCTOR INSTRUCTIONS: _____

_____

_____

_____

ABNORMAL RESULTS: _____

_____

_____

_____

OTHER NOTES: _____

_____

_____

_____

Notes

Medication
List

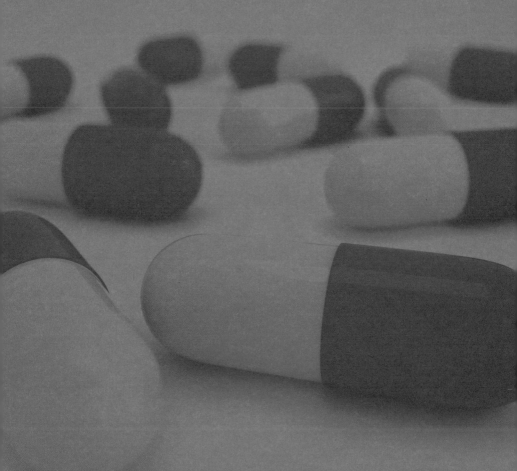

Medication
List

DRUG NAME	DESCRIPTION	DAILY SCHEDULE 2x	
LASix	white oval tablet	TIME	DOSAGE
DOCTOR	**WHY**	8am	4mg
Smith	WATER RETENTION	5pm	4mg
SPECIAL INSTRUCTIONS			
ADVERSE REACTIONS			
DATE STARTED 10/6/2010			
DATE ENDED			

SAMPLE

DRUG NAME	DESCRIPTION	DAILY SCHEDULE 3x	
Insulin	shot	TIME	DOSAGE
DOCTOR	**WHY**	8am	10mg
Smith	Diabetes	12pm	10mg
		5pm	10mg
SPECIAL INSTRUCTIONS 15 mins. before meals			
ADVERSE REACTIONS			
DATE STARTED 10/5/2010			
DATE ENDED			

SAMPLE

DRUG NAME	DESCRIPTION	DAILY SCHEDULE	
		TIME	DOSAGE
DOCTOR	WHY		
SPECIAL INSTRUCTIONS			
ADVERSE REACTIONS			
DATE STARTED			
DATE ENDED			

DRUG NAME	DESCRIPTION	DAILY SCHEDULE	
		TIME	DOSAGE
DOCTOR	WHY		
SPECIAL INSTRUCTIONS			
ADVERSE REACTIONS			
DATE STARTED			
DATE ENDED			

DRUG NAME	DESCRIPTION	DAILY SCHEDULE	
		TIME	DOSAGE
DOCTOR	WHY		
SPECIAL INSTRUCTIONS			
ADVERSE REACTIONS			
DATE STARTED			
DATE ENDED			

DRUG NAME	DESCRIPTION	DAILY SCHEDULE	
		TIME	DOSAGE
DOCTOR	WHY		
SPECIAL INSTRUCTIONS			
ADVERSE REACTIONS			
DATE STARTED			
DATE ENDED			

DRUG NAME	DESCRIPTION	DAILY SCHEDULE	
		TIME	DOSAGE
DOCTOR	WHY		
SPECIAL INSTRUCTIONS			
ADVERSE REACTIONS			
DATE STARTED			
DATE ENDED			

DRUG NAME	DESCRIPTION	DAILY SCHEDULE	
		TIME	DOSAGE
DOCTOR	WHY		
SPECIAL INSTRUCTIONS			
ADVERSE REACTIONS			
DATE STARTED			
DATE ENDED			

DRUG NAME	DESCRIPTION	DAILY SCHEDULE	
		TIME	DOSAGE
DOCTOR	WHY		
SPECIAL INSTRUCTIONS			
ADVERSE REACTIONS			
DATE STARTED			
DATE ENDED			

DRUG NAME	DESCRIPTION	DAILY SCHEDULE	
		TIME	DOSAGE
DOCTOR	WHY		
SPECIAL INSTRUCTIONS			
ADVERSE REACTIONS			
DATE STARTED			
DATE ENDED			

DRUG NAME	DESCRIPTION	DAILY SCHEDULE	
		TIME	DOSAGE
DOCTOR	WHY		
SPECIAL INSTRUCTIONS			
ADVERSE REACTIONS			
DATE STARTED			
DATE ENDED			

DRUG NAME	DESCRIPTION	DAILY SCHEDULE	
		TIME	DOSAGE
DOCTOR	WHY		
SPECIAL INSTRUCTIONS			
ADVERSE REACTIONS			
DATE STARTED			
DATE ENDED			

DRUG NAME	DESCRIPTION	DAILY SCHEDULE	
		TIME	DOSAGE
DOCTOR	WHY		
SPECIAL INSTRUCTIONS			
ADVERSE REACTIONS			
DATE STARTED			
DATE ENDED			

DRUG NAME	DESCRIPTION	DAILY SCHEDULE	
		TIME	DOSAGE
DOCTOR	WHY		
SPECIAL INSTRUCTIONS			
ADVERSE REACTIONS			
DATE STARTED			
DATE ENDED			

DRUG NAME	DESCRIPTION	DAILY SCHEDULE	
		TIME	DOSAGE
DOCTOR	WHY		
SPECIAL INSTRUCTIONS			
ADVERSE REACTIONS			
DATE STARTED			
DATE ENDED			

DRUG NAME	DESCRIPTION	DAILY SCHEDULE	
		TIME	DOSAGE
DOCTOR	WHY		
SPECIAL INSTRUCTIONS			
ADVERSE REACTIONS			
DATE STARTED			
DATE ENDED			

DRUG NAME	DESCRIPTION	DAILY SCHEDULE	
		TIME	DOSAGE
DOCTOR	WHY		
SPECIAL INSTRUCTIONS			
ADVERSE REACTIONS			
DATE STARTED			
DATE ENDED			

DRUG NAME	DESCRIPTION	DAILY SCHEDULE	
		TIME	DOSAGE
DOCTOR	WHY		
SPECIAL INSTRUCTIONS			
ADVERSE REACTIONS			
DATE STARTED			
DATE ENDED			

DRUG NAME	DESCRIPTION	DAILY SCHEDULE	
		TIME	DOSAGE
DOCTOR	WHY		
SPECIAL INSTRUCTIONS			
ADVERSE REACTIONS			
DATE STARTED			
DATE ENDED			

DRUG NAME	DESCRIPTION	DAILY SCHEDULE	
		TIME	DOSAGE
DOCTOR	WHY		
SPECIAL INSTRUCTIONS			
ADVERSE REACTIONS			
DATE STARTED			
DATE ENDED			

DRUG NAME	DESCRIPTION	DAILY SCHEDULE	
		TIME	DOSAGE
DOCTOR	WHY		
SPECIAL INSTRUCTIONS			
ADVERSE REACTIONS			
DATE STARTED			
DATE ENDED			

DRUG NAME	DESCRIPTION	DAILY SCHEDULE	
		TIME	DOSAGE
DOCTOR	WHY		
SPECIAL INSTRUCTIONS			
ADVERSE REACTIONS			
DATE STARTED			
DATE ENDED			

DRUG NAME	DESCRIPTION	DAILY SCHEDULE	
		TIME	DOSAGE
DOCTOR	WHY		
SPECIAL INSTRUCTIONS			
ADVERSE REACTIONS			
DATE STARTED			
DATE ENDED			

Notes

Supplement
List

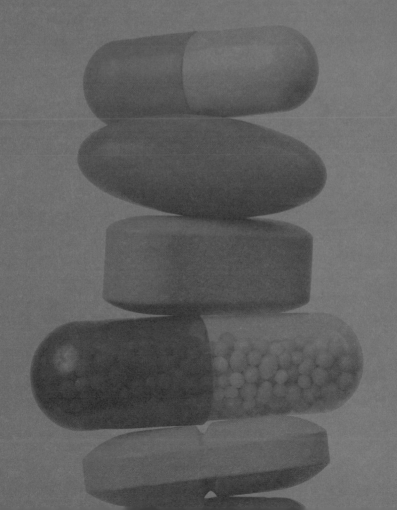

Supplement List

SUPPLEMENT NAME	DESCRIPTION	DAILY SCHEDULE *1x*	
Vitamin D	*yellow gel cap*	**TIME**	**DOSAGE**
DOCTOR	**WHY**	*12pm*	*1,000 IU*
N/A	*bone health*		
SPECIAL INSTRUCTIONS *take with food*			
ADVERSE REACTIONS			
DATE STARTED			
DATE ENDED			

SAMPLE

SUPPLEMENT NAME	DESCRIPTION	DAILY SCHEDULE *1x*	
Multivitamin	*red/orange gummies*	**TIME**	**DOSAGE**
DOCTOR	**WHY**	*9am*	*2 gummies*
N/A	*N/A*		
SPECIAL INSTRUCTIONS			
ADVERSE REACTIONS			
DATE STARTED			
DATE ENDED			

SAMPLE

SUPPLEMENT NAME	DESCRIPTION	DAILY SCHEDULE	
		TIME	DOSAGE
DOCTOR	WHY		
SPECIAL INSTRUCTIONS			
ADVERSE REACTIONS			
DATE STARTED			
DATE ENDED			

SUPPLEMENT NAME	DESCRIPTION	DAILY SCHEDULE	
		TIME	DOSAGE
DOCTOR	WHY		
SPECIAL INSTRUCTIONS			
ADVERSE REACTIONS			
DATE STARTED			
DATE ENDED			

SUPPLEMENT NAME	DESCRIPTION	DAILY SCHEDULE	
		TIME	DOSAGE
DOCTOR	WHY		
SPECIAL INSTRUCTIONS			
ADVERSE REACTIONS			
DATE STARTED			
DATE ENDED			

SUPPLEMENT NAME	DESCRIPTION	DAILY SCHEDULE	
		TIME	DOSAGE
DOCTOR	WHY		
SPECIAL INSTRUCTIONS			
ADVERSE REACTIONS			
DATE STARTED			
DATE ENDED			

SUPPLEMENT NAME	DESCRIPTION	DAILY SCHEDULE	
		TIME	DOSAGE
DOCTOR	WHY		
SPECIAL INSTRUCTIONS			
ADVERSE REACTIONS			
DATE STARTED			
DATE ENDED			

SUPPLEMENT NAME	DESCRIPTION	DAILY SCHEDULE	
		TIME	DOSAGE
DOCTOR	WHY		
SPECIAL INSTRUCTIONS			
ADVERSE REACTIONS			
DATE STARTED			
DATE ENDED			

SUPPLEMENT NAME	DESCRIPTION	DAILY SCHEDULE	
		TIME	DOSAGE
DOCTOR	WHY		
SPECIAL INSTRUCTIONS			
ADVERSE REACTIONS			
DATE STARTED			
DATE ENDED			

SUPPLEMENT NAME	DESCRIPTION	DAILY SCHEDULE	
		TIME	DOSAGE
DOCTOR	WHY		
SPECIAL INSTRUCTIONS			
ADVERSE REACTIONS			
DATE STARTED			
DATE ENDED			

SUPPLEMENT NAME	DESCRIPTION	DAILY SCHEDULE	
		TIME	DOSAGE
DOCTOR	WHY		
SPECIAL INSTRUCTIONS			
ADVERSE REACTIONS			
DATE STARTED			
DATE ENDED			

SUPPLEMENT NAME	DESCRIPTION	DAILY SCHEDULE	
		TIME	DOSAGE
DOCTOR	WHY		
SPECIAL INSTRUCTIONS			
ADVERSE REACTIONS			
DATE STARTED			
DATE ENDED			

SUPPLEMENT NAME	DESCRIPTION	DAILY SCHEDULE	
		TIME	DOSAGE
DOCTOR	WHY		
SPECIAL INSTRUCTIONS			
ADVERSE REACTIONS			
DATE STARTED			
DATE ENDED			

SUPPLEMENT NAME	DESCRIPTION	DAILY SCHEDULE	
		TIME	DOSAGE
DOCTOR	WHY		
SPECIAL INSTRUCTIONS			
ADVERSE REACTIONS			
DATE STARTED			
DATE ENDED			

SUPPLEMENT NAME	DESCRIPTION	DAILY SCHEDULE	
		TIME	DOSAGE
DOCTOR	WHY		
SPECIAL INSTRUCTIONS			
ADVERSE REACTIONS			
DATE STARTED			
DATE ENDED			

SUPPLEMENT NAME	DESCRIPTION	DAILY SCHEDULE	
		TIME	DOSAGE
DOCTOR	WHY		
SPECIAL INSTRUCTIONS			
ADVERSE REACTIONS			
DATE STARTED			
DATE ENDED			

SUPPLEMENT NAME	DESCRIPTION	DAILY SCHEDULE	
		TIME	DOSAGE
DOCTOR	WHY		
SPECIAL INSTRUCTIONS			
ADVERSE REACTIONS			
DATE STARTED			
DATE ENDED			

SUPPLEMENT NAME	DESCRIPTION	DAILY SCHEDULE	
		TIME	DOSAGE
DOCTOR	WHY		
SPECIAL INSTRUCTIONS			
ADVERSE REACTIONS			
DATE STARTED			
DATE ENDED			

SUPPLEMENT NAME	DESCRIPTION	DAILY SCHEDULE	
		TIME	DOSAGE
DOCTOR	WHY		
SPECIAL INSTRUCTIONS			
ADVERSE REACTIONS			
DATE STARTED			
DATE ENDED			

SUPPLEMENT NAME	DESCRIPTION	DAILY SCHEDULE	
		TIME	DOSAGE
DOCTOR	WHY		
SPECIAL INSTRUCTIONS			
ADVERSE REACTIONS			
DATE STARTED			
DATE ENDED			

SUPPLEMENT NAME	DESCRIPTION	DAILY SCHEDULE	
		TIME	DOSAGE
DOCTOR	WHY		
SPECIAL INSTRUCTIONS			
ADVERSE REACTIONS			
DATE STARTED			
DATE ENDED			

SUPPLEMENT NAME	DESCRIPTION	DAILY SCHEDULE	
		TIME	DOSAGE
DOCTOR	WHY		
SPECIAL INSTRUCTIONS			
ADVERSE REACTIONS			
DATE STARTED			
DATE ENDED			

SUPPLEMENT NAME	DESCRIPTION	DAILY SCHEDULE	
		TIME	DOSAGE
DOCTOR	WHY		
SPECIAL INSTRUCTIONS			
ADVERSE REACTIONS			
DATE STARTED			
DATE ENDED			

Notes

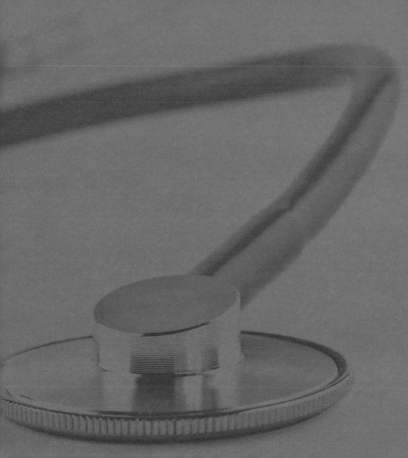

Doctor Contacts

Doctor
Contacts

DOCTOR NAME _____

SPECIALTY: _____

TYPICAL TIME FOR ROUNDS: _____

OFFICE PHONE: _____ CELL PHONE: _____

E-MAIL: _____

OFFICE RECEPTIONIST: _____

NURSE-PRACTITIONER: _____ NP CONTACT INFO: _____

PA: _____ PA CONTACT INFO: _____

HOSPITAL RESIDENT/INTERN REPORTING TO DOCTOR: _____

CONTACT INFO: _____

DOCTOR NAME _____

SPECIALTY: _____

TYPICAL TIME FOR ROUNDS: _____

OFFICE PHONE: _____ CELL PHONE: _____

E-MAIL: _____

OFFICE RECEPTIONIST: _____

NURSE-PRACTITIONER: _____ NP CONTACT INFO: _____

PA: _____ PA CONTACT INFO: _____

HOSPITAL RESIDENT/INTERN REPORTING TO DOCTOR: _____

CONTACT INFO: _____

DOCTOR NAME

SPECIALTY:

TYPICAL TIME FOR ROUNDS:

OFFICE PHONE: CELL PHONE:

E-MAIL:

OFFICE RECEPTIONIST:

NURSE-PRACTITIONER: NP CONTACT INFO:

PA: PA CONTACT INFO:

HOSPITAL RESIDENT/INTERN REPORTING TO DOCTOR:

CONTACT INFO:

DOCTOR NAME

SPECIALTY:

TYPICAL TIME FOR ROUNDS:

OFFICE PHONE: CELL PHONE:

E-MAIL:

OFFICE RECEPTIONIST:

NURSE-PRACTITIONER: NP CONTACT INFO:

PA: PA CONTACT INFO:

HOSPITAL RESIDENT/INTERN REPORTING TO DOCTOR:

CONTACT INFO:

SPECIAL NOTES:

DOCTOR NAME

SPECIALTY:

TYPICAL TIME FOR ROUNDS:

OFFICE PHONE: CELL PHONE:

E-MAIL:

OFFICE RECEPTIONIST:

NURSE-PRACTITIONER: NP CONTACT INFO:

PA: PA CONTACT INFO:

HOSPITAL RESIDENT/INTERN REPORTING TO DOCTOR:

CONTACT INFO:

DOCTOR NAME

SPECIALTY:

TYPICAL TIME FOR ROUNDS:

OFFICE PHONE: CELL PHONE:

E-MAIL:

OFFICE RECEPTIONIST:

NURSE-PRACTITIONER: NP CONTACT INFO:

PA: PA CONTACT INFO:

HOSPITAL RESIDENT/INTERN REPORTING TO DOCTOR:

CONTACT INFO:

SPECIAL NOTES:

DOCTOR NAME

SPECIALTY:

TYPICAL TIME FOR ROUNDS:

OFFICE PHONE: CELL PHONE:

E-MAIL:

OFFICE RECEPTIONIST:

NURSE-PRACTITIONER: NP CONTACT INFO:

PA: PA CONTACT INFO:

HOSPITAL RESIDENT/INTERN REPORTING TO DOCTOR:

CONTACT INFO:

DOCTOR NAME

SPECIALTY:

TYPICAL TIME FOR ROUNDS:

OFFICE PHONE: CELL PHONE:

E-MAIL:

OFFICE RECEPTIONIST:

NURSE-PRACTITIONER: NP CONTACT INFO:

PA: PA CONTACT INFO:

HOSPITAL RESIDENT/INTERN REPORTING TO DOCTOR:

CONTACT INFO:

SPECIAL NOTES:

DOCTOR NAME

Specialty:

Typical Time for Rounds:

Office Phone: Cell Phone:

E-mail:

Office Receptionist:

Nurse-Practitioner: NP Contact Info:

PA: PA Contact Info:

Hospital Resident/Intern Reporting to Doctor:

Contact Info:

DOCTOR NAME

Specialty:

Typical Time for Rounds:

Office Phone: Cell Phone:

E-mail:

Office Receptionist:

Nurse-Practitioner: NP Contact Info:

PA: PA Contact Info:

Hospital Resident/Intern Reporting to Doctor:

Contact Info:

Special Notes:

DOCTOR NAME

SPECIALTY:

TYPICAL TIME FOR ROUNDS:

OFFICE PHONE: CELL PHONE:

E-MAIL:

OFFICE RECEPTIONIST:

NURSE-PRACTITIONER: NP CONTACT INFO:

PA: PA CONTACT INFO:

HOSPITAL RESIDENT/INTERN REPORTING TO DOCTOR:

CONTACT INFO:

DOCTOR NAME

SPECIALTY:

TYPICAL TIME FOR ROUNDS:

OFFICE PHONE: CELL PHONE:

E-MAIL:

OFFICE RECEPTIONIST:

NURSE-PRACTITIONER: NP CONTACT INFO:

PA: PA CONTACT INFO:

HOSPITAL RESIDENT/INTERN REPORTING TO DOCTOR:

CONTACT INFO:

SPECIAL NOTES:

Notes

Resources

Resources

Drug and Supplement Facts and Information

While this list is not exhaustive, these online sources represent some of the most reliable and user-friendly repositories for up-to-date and comprehensive information pertaining to medications, supplements, and how they interact with one another.

Physician Desk Reference
www.pdr.net

A comprehensive resource of all prescription medications as well as side effects, drug interactions, and adverse drug reactions. Encyclopedic in scope, it is a reference that many physicians utilize in their daily practice.

Drugs.com
www.drugs.com

A great online resource for information on medications, side effects, and medication interactions. There are sections concerning medical conferences and even a section on natural supplements.

Drug Interaction Checker
www.webmd.com/interaction-checker

This part of WebMD allows you to type in a medication, and the site will bring up medications that interact with it. In addition, you can type in a natural supplement or herb and see which medications, if any, will interact with that substance.

Natural Medicines Comprehensive Database
naturaldatabase.therapeuticresearch.com

This is one of the most comprehensive information sources for herbs and natural supplements. It will give you the latest studies supporting the use of various natural supplements for health conditions. It also includes information concerning medication-herbal interactions. You only need to pay a nominal annual fee for complete access. It is a tremendous information source, and I cannot recommend it highly enough.

Pharmacogenetic Testing

While you can directly obtain this type of testing from the companies below, we urge you to speak with your physician or health-care professional first. Personalized testing needs to be discussed in the context of your own personal health situation. There is no one better to have this discussion with than your physician.

SGS Life Science Services
www.sgs.com/en/life-sciences
This international company performs an extremely wide range of services, including pharmacokinetic testing and metabolic profiling.

LGC Group
www.lgcgroup.com/genomics
With offices in Boston, Kentucky, and all over the globe, this company provides a wide range of genetics testing and measurement services.

Renaissance RX
http://www.renrx.com/
This New Orleans–based company provides services for patients and healthcare providers, including pharmacogenetic and advanced toxicology testing.

General Health Websites

There are a variety of online resources that offer guidelines and summarize the results of the most recent findings related to many health conditions and medications. Here are some of the most authoritative and user-friendly sources:

MedlinePlus
www.nlm.nih.gov/medlineplus/

American Heart Association
www.heart.org

U.S. Food and Drug Administration
www.fda.gov

National Institute of Mental Health
www.nimh.nih.gov/index.shtml

Practical Pain Management
www.practicalpainmanagement.com

NPS MedicineWise
www.nps.org.au

PubMed.gov
www.ncbi.nlm.nih.gov/pubmed/

References

Introduction

Bailey, R.L. et al. "Dietary Supplement Use in the United States, 2003–2006." *Journal of Nutrition* 141, no. 2 (2011): 261–66.

Fan, W. et al. "Pharmacogenetics-Guided Individualized Warfarin Dosing in a Cardiology Clinic." Poster presentation at the nineteenth World Congress on Heart Disease, July 2014.

Mahler, Robert L. et al. "Clinical Consequences of Polypharmacy in Elderly." *Expert Opinion on Drug Safety* 13, no. 1 (Jan. 2014): 57.

Miguel, A. et al. "Frequency of Adverse Drug Reactions in Hospitalized Patients: A Systematic Review and Meta-Analysis." *Pharmacoepidemiology and Drug Safety* 21, no. 11 (July 2012): 1139–54.

Patel, P. et al. "Drug Related Visits to the ER: How Big Is the Problem?" *Pharmacotherapy: The Journal of Human Pharmacology and Drug Therapy* 22 no. 7 (2002): 915–23.

Williams, C.D. et al. "Prevalence of Nonalcoholic Fatty Liver Disease and Nonalcoholic Steatohepatitis among a Largely Middle-Aged Population Utilizing Ultrasound and Liver Biopsy: A Prospective Study." *Gastroenterology* 140, no. 1 (Jan. 2011): 124–31.

Checklist 1

Colombo, D., and G. Bellia. "Cyclosporine and Herbal Supplement Interactions." *Journal of Toxicology* 2014 (2014): Article ID 145325.

NPS MedicineWise. "Mixing Grapefruit with Medicines." *Medicinewise Living* (July 18, 2014). http://www.nps.org.au/publications/consumer/medicinewise-living/2012/mixing-grapefruit-with-medicines.

Checklist 2

Banach, M. et al. "Statin Therapy and Plasma Coenzyme Q_{10} Concentrations–A Systematic Review and Meta-Analysis of Placebo-Controlled Trials." *Pharmacological Research* 99 (Sep. 2015): 329–36.

Castellote, J. et al. "Serious Drug-Induced Liver Disease Secondary to Ezetimibe." *World Journal of Gastroenterology* 14, no. 32 (Aug. 28, 2008): 5098–9.

Elshazly, M.B. et al. "Non-High-Density Lipoprotein Cholesterol, Guideline Targets, and Population Percentiles for Secondary Prevention in 1.3 Million Adults: The VLDL-2 Study (Very Large Database of Lipids)." *Journal of the American College of Cardiology* 62, no. 21 (Nov. 19, 2013): 1960–5.

Florentin, M. et al. "Ezetimibe-Associated Adverse Effects: What the Clinician Needs to Know." *International Journal of Clinical Practice* 62, no. 1 (Jan. 2008): 88–96.

Gillett, R.C., and A. Norrell. "Considerations for Safe Use of Statins: Liver Enzyme Abnormalities and Muscle Toxicity." *American Family Physician* 83, no. 6 (Mar. 15, 2011): 711–6.

Kosoglou, T. et al. "Ezetimibe: A Review of Its Metabolism, Pharmacokinetics and Drug Interactions." *Clinical Pharmacokinetics* 44, no. 5 (2005): 467–94.

Kota, S.K. et al. "Efficacy and Safety of Statin and Fibrate Combination Therapy in Lipid Management." *Diabetes and Metabolic Syndrome* 6, no. 3 (Jul.–Sep. 2012): 173–4.

Li, D.Q. et al. "Risk of Adverse Events among Older Adults Following Co-Prescription of Clarithromycin and Statins Not Metabolized by Cytochrome P450 3A4." *Canadian Medical Association Journal* 187, no. 3 (Feb. 17, 2015): 174–80.

McKenney, J.M. et al. "Safety and Efficacy of Long-Term Co-Administration of Fenofibrate and Ezetimibe in Patients with Mixed Hyperlipidemia." *Journal of the American College of Cardiology* 47, no. 8 (Apr. 18, 2006): 1584–7.

Patel, A.M. et al. "Statin Toxicity from Macrolide Antibiotic Coprescription: A Population-Based Cohort Study." *Annals of Internal Medicine* 158, no. 12 (Jun. 18, 2013): 869–76.

Preiss, D. "The New Pooled Cohort Equations Risk Calculator." *Canadian Journal of Cardiology* 31, no. 5 (May 2015): 613–9.

Sahebkar, A. et al. "New LDL-Cholesterol Lowering Therapies: Pharmacology, Clinical Trials, and Relevance to Acute Coronary Syndromes." *Clinical Therapeutics* 35, no. 8 (Aug. 2013): 1082–98.

Schirris, T.J. et al. "Statin-Induced Myopathy Is Associated with Mitochondrial Complex III Inhibition." *Cell Metabolism* 22, no. 3 (Sep. 1, 2015): 399–407.

Seidah, N.G. "Proprotein Convertase Subtilisin Kexin 9 (PCSK9) Inhibitors in the Treatment of Hypercholesterolemia and Other Pathologies." *Current Pharmaceutical Design* 19, no. 17 (2013): 3161–72.

Slim, H. et al. "Ezetimibe-Related Myopathy: A Systematic Review." *Journal of Clinical Lipidology* 2, no. 5 (Oct. 2008): 328–34.

Checklist 3

Agrawal, S. et al. "Heart Failure and Chronic Kidney Disease: Should We Use Spironolactone?" *American Journal of the Medical Sciences* 350, no. 2 (Aug. 2015): 147–51.

Anderson, J.L. et al. "2012 ACCF/AHA Focused Update Incorporated into the ACCF/AHA 2007 Guidelines for the Management of Patients with Unstable Angina/Non-ST-Elevation Myocardial Infarction: A Report of the American College of Cardiology Foundation/American Heart Association Task Force on Practice Guidelines." *Circulation* 127, no. 23 (2013): e663–e828.

Braunwald, E. et al. "ACC/AHA 2002 Guideline Update for the Management of Patients With Unstable Angina and Non-ST-Segment Elevation Myocardial Infarction - Summary Article: A Report of the American College of Cardiology/American Heart Association Task Force on Practice Guidelines (Committee on the Management of Patients With Unstable Angina)." *Journal of the American College of Cardiology* 40, no. 7 (2002): 1366–74.

Cheitlin, M.D. et al. "ACC/AHA Expert Consensus Document. Use of Sildenafil (Viagra) in Patients With Cardiovascular Disease. American College of Cardiology/American Heart Association." *Journal of American College Cardiology* 33, no. 1 (1999): 273–82.

Fihn, S.D. et al. "2012 ACCF/AHA/ACP/AATS/PCNA/SCAI/STS Guideline for the Diagnosis and Management of Patients With Stable Ischemic Heart Disease: A Report of the American College of Cardiology Foundation/American Heart Association Task Force on Practice Guidelines, and the American College of Physicians, American Association for Thoracic Surgery, Preventive Cardiovascular Nurses Association, Society for Cardiovascular Angiography and Interventions, and Society of Thoracic Surgeons." *Circulation* 126, no. 25 (2012): 3097–137.

Gunasekara, N.S., and S. Noble. "Isosorbide 5-Mononitrate—A Review of a Sustained-Release Formulation (Imdur) in Stable Angina Pectoris." *Drugs* 57, no. 2 (1999): 261–77.

Guo, H. et al. "Clinical Efficacy of Spironolactone for Resistant Hypertension: A Meta Analysis from Randomized Controlled Clinical Trials." *International Journal of Clinical and Experimental Medicine* 8, no. 5 (May 15, 2015): 7270–8.

Haymore, B.R. et al. "Risk of Angioedema with Angiotensin Receptor Blockers in Patients with Prior Angioedema Associated with Angiotensin-Converting Enzyme Inhibitors: A Meta-Analysis." *Annals of Allergy, Asthma, and Immunology* 101, no. 5 (Nov. 2008): 495.

Hester, W. et al. "Thromboprophylaxis with Fondaparinux in High-Risk Postoperative Patients with Renal Insufficiency." *Thrombosis Research* 133, no. 4 (Apr. 2014): 629–33.

James, P.A. et al. "2014 Evidence-Based Guideline for the Management of High Blood Pressure in Adults: Report from the Panel Members Appointed to the Eighth Joint National Committee (JNC 8)." *JAMA* 311, no. 5 (2014): 507–20.

Lin, T.T. et al. "Class Effect of Beta-Blockers in Survivors of ST-Elevation Myocardial Infarction: A Nationwide Cohort Study Using an Insurance Claims Database." *Scientific Reports* 5 (Sep. 2, 2015): 13692.

Loftus, P.A. et al. "Risk Factors Associated with Severe and Recurrent Angioedema: An Epidemic Linked to ACE-Inhibitors." *Laryngoscope* 124, no. 11 (Nov. 2014): 2502–7.

Maack, C. et al. "Beta-Blocker Treatment of Chronic Heart Failure: Comparison of Carvedilol and Metoprolol." *Congestive Heart Failure* 9, no. 5 (Sep.–Oct. 2003): 263–70.

McEvoy, G.K., ed *AHFS® Drug Information, 56th Edition.* Bethesda, MD: American Society of Health-System Pharmacists, 2015.

Michel, T., and B.B. Hoffman. "Chapter 27: Treatment of Myocardial Ischemia and Hypertension." In: *Goodman & Gilman's The Pharmacological Basis of Therapeutics, 12th Edition*, eds. Brunton, L.L., B.A. Chabner, and B.C. Knollmann. New York: McGraw-Hill, 2011.

Narula, H.S. et al. "Gynecomastia—Pathophysiology, Diagnosis and Treatment." *Nature Reviews Endocrinology* 10, no. 11 (Nov. 2014): 684–98.

Saseen, J.J., and E.J. MacLaughlin. "Chapter 3: Hypertension." In: *Pharmacotherapy: A Pathophysiologic Approach, 9th Edition*, eds. J.T. DiPiro et al. New York: McGraw-Hill, 2014.

Sato, A., and S. Fukuda. "A Prospective Study of Frequency and Characteristics of Cough During ACE-Inhibitor Treatment." *Clinical and Experimental Hypertension* 37, no. 7 (Aug. 19, 2015): 1–6.

Schmidt, G.R., and A.A. Schuna. "Rebound Hypertension After Discontinuation of Transdermal Clonidine." *Clinical Pharmacy* 7, no. 10 (Oct. 1988): 772–4.

Wodlinger Jackson, A.M. "Chapter 5: Cardiovascular Agents." *Frequently Prescribed Medications: Drugs You Need to Know, 2nd Edition*, eds. Mancano, Michael A., and Jason C.

Gallagher. Burlington, VT: Jones & Bartlett Learning, 2014.

Checklist 4

Abrams, P.J., and C.R. Emerson. "Rivaroxaban: A Novel, Oral, Direct Factor Xa Inhibitor." *Pharmacotherapy* 29, no. 2 (2009): 167–81.

Alban, S. "Pharmacological Strategies for Inhibition of Thrombin Activity." *Current Pharmaceutical Design* 14, no. 12 (2008): 1152–75.

Hobl, E.L. et al. "Morphine Decreases Clopidogrel Concentrations and Effects: A Randomized, Double-Blind, Placebo-Controlled Trial." *Journal of the American College of Cardiology* 63, no.7 (Feb. 25, 2014): 630–5.

Hobl, E.L. et al. "Morphine Interaction with Prasugrel: A Double-Blind, Cross-Over Trial in Healthy Volunteers." *Clinical Research in Cardiology.* Published electronically Oct. 22, 2015.

January, C.T. et al. "2014 AHA/ACC/HRS Guideline for the Management of Patients with Atrial Fibrillation: A Report of the American College of Cardiology/American Heart Association Task Force on Practice Guidelines and the Heart Rhythm Society." *Circulation* 130, no. 23 (2014): e199–e267.

Khalighi, K. et al. "CYP2D6 Genetic Information-Guided Metoprolol Use in a Cardiology Clinic—A Prospective Study." Poster presented at the Heart Rhythm Society, Boston, MA: 2015.

Khalighi, K. et al. "Genetic Information-Guided Thromboembolism Precaution and Treatment in a Cardiology Clinic—A Prospective Study." Poster presented at the Heart Rhythm Society, Boston, MA: 2015.

Khalighi, K. et al. "Pharmacogenetics-Guided Individual Warfarin Dosing—A Prospective Observatory Study." Poster presented at the Heart Rhythm Society, Boston, MA: 2015.

Kubika, J. et al. "Morphine Delays and Attenuates Ticagrelor Exposure and Action in Patients with Myocardial Infarction: The Randomized, Double-Blind, Placebo-Controlled IMPRESSION Trial." *European Heart Journal.* Published electronically Oct. 21, 2015.

Pollack, Charles V. et al. "Idarucizumab for Dabigatran Reversal." *New England Journal of Medicine* 373 (Aug. 6, 2015): 511–20.

Wodlinger Jackson, A.M. "Chapter 5: Cardiovascular Agents." *Frequently Prescribed Medications: Drugs You Need to Know, 2nd Edition,* eds. Mancano, Michael A., and Jason C. Gallagher. Burlington, MA: Jones & Bartlett Learning: 2014,

Checklist 5

Baumann, P. "Pharmacokinetic-Pharmacodynamic Relationship of the Selective Serotonin Reuptake Inhibitors." *Clinical Pharmacokinetics* 31, no.6 (Dec. 1996): 444–69.

Beakley, B.D. et al. "Tramadol, Pharmacology, Side Effects, and Serotonin Syndrome: A Review." *Pain Physician* 18, no. 4 (Jul.–Aug. 2015): 395–400.

de Braqanca, A.C. et al. "Carbamazepine Can Induce Kidney Water Absorption by Increasing Aquaporin 2 Expression." *Nephrology Dialysis and Transplantation* 25, no. 12 (Dec. 2010): 3840–5.

deLeon, J. et al. "The CYP2D6 Poor Metabolizer Phenotype May Be Associated with Risperidone Adverse Drug Reactions and Discontinuation." *Journal of Clinical Psychiatry* 66, no. 1 (Jan. 2005): 15–27.

Edwardsson, B. "Venlafaxine as Single Therapy Associated with Hypertensive Encephalopathy." *Springerplus* 4 (Feb. 26, 2015): 97.

Grossman, A. et al. "Drug Induced Hypertension—An Unappreciated Cause of Secondary Hypertension." *European Journal of Pharmacology* 763 (Jun. 19, 2015): 15–22.

Grunebaum, M.F. et al. "SSRI Versus Bupropion Effects on Symptom Clusters in Suicidal Depression: Post Hoc Analysis of a Randomized Clinical Trial." *Journal of Clinical Psychiatry* 74, no. 9 (Sep. 2013): 872–9.

Gupta, E. et al. "Severe Hyponatremia Due to Valproic Acid Toxicity." *Journal of Clinical Medicine Research* 7, no. 9 (Sep. 2015): 717–9.

Härtter, S. et al. "Differential Effects of Fluvoxamine and Other Antidepressants on the Biotransformation of Melatonin." *Journal of*

Clinical Psychopharmacology 21, no. 2 (Apr. 2001): 167–74.

Hirsh-Rokrach, B. et al. "Differential Impact of Selective Serotonin Reuptake Inhibitors on Platelet Response to Clopidogrel: A Randomized, Double-Blind, Crossover Trial." *Pharmacotherapy* 35, no. 2 (Feb. 2015): 140–7.

Imam, S.H. et al. "Free Phenytoin Toxicity." *American Journal of Emergency Medicine* 32, no. 10 (Oct. 2014): 1301.e3–4.

Iqbal, M.M. et al. "Overview of Serotonin Syndrome." *Annals of Clinical Psychiatry* 24, no. 4 (Nov. 2012): 310–8.

Kaufman, K.R. et al. "Myoclonus in Renal Failure: Two Cases of Gabapentin Toxicity." *Epilepsy and Behavior Case Reports* 2 (Dec. 29, 2013): 8–10.

Krishnamoorthy, G. et al. "Early Predisposition to Osteomalacia in Indian Adults on Phenytoin or Valproate Monotherapy and Effective Prophylaxis by Simultaneous Supplementation with Calcium and 25-Hydroxy Vitamin D at Recommended Daily Allowance Dosage: A Prospective Study." *Neurology India* 58, no. 2 (Mar.–Apr. 2010): 213–9.

Lal, R. et al. "Clinical Pharmacokinetics of Gabapentin after Administration of Gabapentin Enacarbil Extended-Release Tablets in Patients with Varying Degrees of Renal Function Using Data from an Open-Label, Single-Dose Pharmacokinetic Study." *Clinical Therapeutics* 34, no. 1 (Jan. 2012): 201–13.

Launiainen, T. et al. "Fatal Venlafaxine Poisonings Are Associated with a High Prevalence of Drug Interactions." *International Journal of Legal Medicine* 125, no. 3 (May 2011): 349–58

Lazzari, A.A. et al. "Prevention of Bone Loss and Vertebral Fractures in Patients with Chronic Epilepsy–Antiepileptic Drug and Osteoporosis Prevention Trial." *Epilepsia* 54, no. 11 (Nov. 2013): 1997–2004.

Makris, G.D. et al. "Serotonergic Medication Enhances the Association Between Suicide and Sunshine." *Journal of Affective Disorders* 189 (Jan. 1, 2016): 276–281.

Michaelets, E.L. "Update: Clinically Significant Cytochrome P-450 Drug Interactions." *Pharmacotherapy* 18, no. 1 (1998): 84–112.

Mintzer, S. et al. "Vitamin D Levels and Bone Turnover in Epilepsy Patients Taking Carbamazepine or Oxcarbazepine." *Epilepsia* 47, no. 3 (Mar. 2006): 510–5.

Montejo-Gonzalez, A.L. et al. "SSRI-Induced Sexual Dysfunction: Fluoxetine, Paroxetine, Sertraline, and Fluvoxamine in a Prospective, Multicenter, and Descriptive Clinical Study of 344 Patients." *Journal of Sex and Marital Therapy* 23, no. 3 (Fall 1997): 176–94.

Probst-Schendzielorz, K. et al. "Effect of Cytochrome P450 Polymorphism on the Action and Metabolism of Selective Serotonin Reuptake Inhibitors." *Expert Opinion and Drug Metabolism and Toxicology* 11, no. 8 (Aug. 2015): 1219–32.

Schwartz, A.R. et al. "Dextromethorphan-Induced Serotonin Syndrome." *Clinical Toxicology* 46, no. 8 (Sep. 2008): 771–3.

Stevens, D.L. "Association Between Selective Serotonin-Reuptake Inhibitors, Second-Generation Antipsychotics, and Neuroleptic Malignant Syndrome." *The Annals of Pharmacotherapy* 42, no. 9 (Sep. 2008): 1290–7.

Sun-Edelstein, C. et al. "Drug-Induced Serotonin Syndrome: A Review." *Expert Opinion on Drug Safety* 7, no. 5 (Sep. 2008): 587–96.

Von Wincklemann, S.L. et al. "Therapeutic Drug Monitoring of Phenytoin in Critically Ill Patients. *Pharmacotherapy* 28, no. 11 (Nov. 2008): 1391–400.

Wellington, K. et al. "Oxcarbazepine: An Update of Its Efficacy in the Management of Epilepsy." *CNS Drugs* 15, no. 2 (2001): 137–63.

Wooltorton, E. "Bupropion (Zyban, Wellbutrin SR): Reports of Deaths, Seizures, Serum Sickness." *Canadian Medical Association Journal* 166, no. 1 (Jan 8. 2002): 68.

Zhang, L.L. et al. "Side Effects of Phenobarbital in Epilepsy: A Systematic Review." *Epileptic Disorders* 13, no. 4 (Dec. 2011): 349–65.

Zhou, S. et al. "Pharmacokinetic Interactions of Drugs with St. John's Wort." *Journal of Psychopharmacology* 18, no. 2 (Jun. 2004): 262–76.

Checklist 6

Billington, E.O. et al. "The Effect of Thiazolidinediones on Bone Mineral Density and Bone Turnover: Systematic Review and Meta-Analysis." *Diabetologia* 58, no. 10 (Oct. 2015): 2238–46.

Blonde, L. et al. "Gastrointestinal Tolerability of Extended-Release Metformin Tablets Compared to Immediate-Release Metformin Tablets: Results of a Retrospective Cohort Study." *Current Medical Research and Opinion* 20, no. 4 (Apr. 2004): 565–72.

Boerner, Brian, Clifford D Miles, and Vijay Shivaswamy. "Efficacy and Safety of Sitagliptin for the Treatment of New-Onset Diabetes After Renal Transplantation." *International Journal of Endocrinology* 2014 (2014): 617638.

Brown, N.J. et al. "Dipeptidyl Peptidase-IV Inhibitor Use Associated with Increased Risk of ACE Inhibitor-Associated Angioedema." *Hypertension* 54, no. 3 (Sep. 2009): 516–23.

Byrd, J.S. et al. "DPP-4 Inhibitors and Angioedema: A Cause for Concern?" *Annals of Allergy, Asthma and Immunology* 106, no. 5 (May 2011): 436–8.

Chitturi, S., and George, J. "Hepatotoxicity of Commonly Used Drugs: Nonsteroidal Anti-Inflammatory Drugs, Antihypertensives, Antidiabetic Agents, Anticonvulsants, Lipid-Lowering Agents, Psychotropic Drugs." *Seminars in Liver Disease* 22, no. 2 (2002): 169–83.

Colmers, I.N. et al. "Use of Thiazolidinediones and the Risk of Bladder Cancer among People with Type 2 Diabetes: A Meta-Analysis." *Canadian Medical Association Journal* 184, no. 12 (Sep. 4, 2012): E675–83.

Dujic, T. et al. "Organic Cation Transporter 1 Variants and Gastrointestinal Side Effects of Metformin in Patients with Type 2 Diabetes." *Diabetic Medicine.* Published electronically Nov. 25, 2015.

Elmore, L.K. et al. "A Review of the Efficacy and Safety of Canagliflozin in Elderly Patients with Type 2 Diabetes." *The Consultant Pharmacist* 29, no. 5 (2014): 335–46.

Erondu, N. et al. "Diabetic Ketoacidosis and Related Events in the Canagliflozin Type 2

Diabetes Clinical Program." *Diabetes Care* 38, no. 9 (Jul. 22, 2015): 1680–6.

Hinnen, D. "Glucuretic Effects and Renal Safety of Dapagliflozin in Patients with Type 2 Diabetes." *Therapeutic Advances in Endocrinology and Metabolism* 6, no. 3 (Jun. 2015): 92–102.

Horita, S. et al. "Thiazolidinediones and Edema: Recent Advances in the Pathogenesis of Thiazolidinediones-Induced Renal Sodium Retention." *PPAR Research* 2015 (2015): Article ID 646423.

Johnson, N.P. "Metformin Use in Women with Polycystic Ovary Syndrome." *Annals of Translational Medicine* 2, no. 6 (Jun. 2014): 56.

Kahn, C.R. et al. "Unraveling the Mechanism of Action of Thiazolidinediones." *Journal of Clinical Investigation* 106, no. 11 (Dec. 2000): 1305–7.

Lewis, J.D. et al. "Risk of Bladder Cancer Among Diabetic Patients Treated with Pioglitazone: Interim Report of a Longitudinal Cohort Study." *Diabetic Care* 34, no. 4 (Apr. 2011): 916–22.

Li, J. et al. "Troglitazone Enhances the Hepatotoxicity of Acetaminophen by Inducing CYP3A in Rats." *Toxicology* 176, nos. 1–2 (Jul. 1, 2002): 91–100.

Luong, D.Q. et al. "Metformin Treatment Improves Weight and Dyslipidemia in Children with Metabolic Syndrome." *Journal of Pediatric Endocrinology and Metabolism* 28, nos. 5–6 (May 2015): 649–55.

MacConell, L. et al. "Safety and Tolerability of Exenatide Once Weekly in Patients with Type 2 Diabetes: An Integrated Analysis of 4,328 Patients." *Diabetes Metabolic Syndrome and Obesity* 8 (May 18, 2015): 241–53.

Micheli, L. et al. "Severe Hypoglycemia Associated with Levofloxacin in Type 2 Diabetic Patients Receiving Polytherapy: Two Case Reports." *International Journal of Clinical Pharmacology and Therapeutics* 50, no. 4 (Apr. 2012): 302–6.

Parra, D. et al. "Metformin Monitoring and Change in Serum Creatinine Levels in Patients Undergoing Radiologic Procedures Involving Administration of Intravenous Contrast Media." *Pharmacotherapy* 24, no. 8 (Aug. 2004): 987–93.

Prasad-Reddy, L. et al. "A Clinical Review of GLP-1 Receptor Agonists: Efficacy and Safety in Diabetes and Beyond." *Drugs in Context* 4 (Jul. 9, 2015): Article ID 212283.

Scheen, A.J. "Drug-Drug Interactions with Sodium-Glucose Cotransporters Type 2 (SGLT2) Inhibitors, New Oral Glucose-Lowering Agents for the Management of Type 2 Diabetes Mellitus." *Clinical Pharmacokinetics* 53, no. 4 (Apr. 2014): 295–304.

Scheen, A.J. "Pharmacokinetics and Clinical Use of Incretin-Based Therapies in Patients with Chronic Kidney Disease and Type 2 Diabetes." *Clinical Pharmacokinetics* 54, no. 1 (Jan. 2015): 1–21.

Schneeberger, C. et al. "Asymptomatic Bacteriuria and Urinary Tract Infections in Special Patient Groups: Women with Diabetes Mellitus and Pregnant Women." *Current Opinion in Infectious Disease* 27, no. 1 (Feb. 2014): 108–14.

Snyder, R.W., and J.S. Berns. "Use of Insulin and Oral Hypoglycemic Medications in Patients with Diabetes Mellitus and Advanced Kidney Disease." *Seminars in Dialysis* 17, no. 5 (Sep.-Oct. 2004): 365–70.

St. Peter, J.V. et al. "Factors Associated with the Risk of Liver Enzyme Elevation in Patients with Type 2 Diabetes Treated with a Thiazolidinedione." *Pharmacotherapy* 21, no. 2 (Feb. 2001): 183–8.

Thompson, A.M. et al. "Dulaglutide: The Newest GLP-1 Receptor Agonist for the Management of Type 2 Diabetes." *The Annals of Pharmacotherapy* 49, no. 3 (Mar. 2015): 351–9.

Turner, R.M. et al. "Thiazolidinediones and Associated Risk of Bladder Cancer: A Systematic Review and Meta-Analysis." *British Journal of Clinical Pharmacology* 78, no. 2 (Aug. 2014): 258–73.

Xu, T. et al. "Effects of Metformin on Metabolite Profiles and LDL Cholesterol in Patients with Type 2 Diabetes." *Diabetes Care* 38, no. 10 (Oct. 2015).

Vangoitsenhoven, R. et al. "GLP1 and Cancer: Friend or Foe?" *Endocrine Related Cancer* 19, no. 5 (Sep. 5, 2012): F77–88.

Young, M.A. et al. "Coadministration of Acetaminophen and Troglitazone: Pharmacokinetics and Safety." *Journal of Clinical Pharmacology* 38, no. 9 (Sep. 1998): 819–24.

Zhu, Z. et al. "Increased Risk of Bladder Cancer with Pioglitazone Therapy in Patients with Diabetes: A Meta-Analysis." *Diabetes Research and Clinical Practice* 98, no. 1 (Oct. 2012): 159–63.

Zhu, Z. et al. "Risk of Fracture with Thiazolidinediones: An Updated Meta-Analysis of Randomized Clinical Trials." *Bone* 68 (Nov. 2014): 115–23.

Checklist 7

Barletta, J.F. et al. "Proton Pump Inhibitors Increase the Risk for Hospital-Acquired Clostridium Difficile Infection in Critically Ill Patients." *Critical Care* 18, no. 6 (Dec. 24, 2014): 714.

Cole, S.A., and T.J. Stahl. "Persistent and Recurrent *Clostridium difficile* Colitis." *Clinics in Colon and Rectal Surgery* 28, no. 2 (Jun. 2015): 65–9.

Dhir, R., and J.E. Richter. "Erythromycin in the Short- and Long-Term Control of Dyspepsia Symptoms in Patients with Gastroparesis." *Journal of Clinical Gastroenterology* 38, no. 3 (Mar. 2004): 237–42.

Fedorowicz, Z., E.J. van Zuuren, and N. Hu. "Histamine H2-Receptor Antagonists for Urticaria." *Cochrane Database of Systematic Reviews* 3 (Mar. 14, 2012).

Fish, D.N. "Fluoroquinolone Adverse Effects and Drug Interactions." *Pharmacotherapy* 21, no. 10 (Oct. 2001): 253–272.

Fisher, R.S. "Sucralfate: A Review of Drug Tolerance and Safety." *Journal of Clinical Gastroenterology* 3, suppl. 2 (1981): 181–4.

Freedburg, D.E. et al. "Use of Proton Pump Inhibitors Is Associated with Fractures in Young Adults: A Population-Based Study." *Osteoporosis International* 26, no. 10 (Oct. 2015): 2501–7.

Foti, C. et al. "Hypersensitivity Reaction to Ranitidine: Description of a Case and Review of the Literature." *Immunopharmacology and Immunotoxicology* 31, no. 3 (2009): 414–6.

Gurevitz, S.L. "Erythromycin: Drug Interactions." *Journal of Dental Hygiene* 71, no. 4 (Summer 1997): 159–61.

Heidelbaugh, J.J. "Proton Pump Inhibitors and Risk of Vitamin and Mineral Deficiency: Evidence and Clinical Implications." *Therapeutic Advances in Drug Safety* 4, no. 3 (Jun. 2013): 125–33.

Ishimori, A. "Safety Experience with Sucralfate in Japan." *Journal of Clinical Gastroenterology* 3, suppl. 2 (1981): 169–73.

Knodell, R.G. et al. "Differential Inhibition of Individual Human Liver Cytochromes P-450 by Cimetidine." *Gastroenterology* 101, no. 6 (1991): 1680–91.

Liu, N.N., and J.R. Köhler. "Antagonism of Fluconazole and a Proton Pump Inhibitor Against *Candida albicans*." *Antimicrobal Agents and Chemotherapy*. Published electronically Nov. 23, 2015.

Miller, S.J. "Medication-Nutrient Interactions: Hypophosphatemia Associated with Sucralfate in the Intensive Care Unit." *Nutrition in Clinical Practice* 6, no. 5 (1991): 199–201

Moberg, L.M. et al. "Use of Proton Pump Inhibitors (PPI) and History of Earlier Fracture Are Independent Risk Factors for Fracture in Postmenopausal Women. The WHILA study." *Maturitas* 78, no. 4 (Aug. 2014): 310–5.

Parkman, H.P. et al. "Metoclopramide Nasal Spray Is Effective in Symptoms of Gastroparesis in Diabetics Compared to Conventional Oral Tablet." *Neurogastroenterology and Motility* 26, no. 4 (Apr. 2014): 521–8.

Parkman, H.P. et al. "Metoclopramide Nasal Spray Reduces Symptoms of Gastroparesis in Women, but Not Men, with Diabetes: Results of a Phase 2B Randomized Study." *Clinical Gastroenterology and Hepatology* 13, no. 7 (Jul. 2015): 1256–63.

Sax, M.J. "Clinically Important Adverse Effects and Drug Interactions with H2-Receptor Antagonists: An Update." *Pharmacotherapy* 7, no. 6 (1987): 110S–15S.

Shikata, T. et al. "Use of Proton Pump Inhibitors Is Associated with Anemia in Cardiovascular Outpatients." *Circulation Journal* 79, no. 1 (2015): 193–200.

Smith, R., and M.J. Kendall. "Ranitidine Versus Cimetidine. A Comparison of Their Potential to Cause Clinically Important Drug Interactions." *Clinical Pharmacokinetics* 15, no. 1 (Jul. 1988): 44–56.

Suzuki, K., et al. "Co-Administration of Proton Pump Inhibitors Delays Elimination of Plasma Methotrexate in High-Dose Methotrexate Therapy." *British Journal of Clinical Pharmacology* 67, no. 1 (Jan. 2009): 44–9.

von Rosensteil, N.A., and D. Adam. "Macrolide Antibacterials. Drug Interactions of Clinical Significance." *Drug Safety* 13, no. 2 (Aug. 1995): 105–22.

Wysowski, D.K. et al. "Postmarketing Reports of QT Prolongation and Ventricular Arrhythmia in Association with Cisapride and Food and Drug Administration Regulatory Actions." *American Journal of Gastroenterology* 96, no. 6 (Jun. 2001): 1698–703.

Checklist 8

Ajadhey, H. et al. "Comparative Effects of Non-Steroidal Anti-Inflammatory Drugs (NSAIDs) on Blood Pressure in Patients with Hypertension." *BMC Cardiovascular Disorders* 12 (Oct. 24, 2012): 93.

Bell, A.J., and G. Duggin. "Acute Methyl Salicylate Toxicity Complicating Herbal Skin Treatment for Psoriasis." *Emergency Medicine* 14, no. 2 (Jun. 2002): 188–90.

Cepedad, M.S. et al. "Tramadol for Osteoarthritis: A Systematic Review and Meta Analysis." *Journal of Rheumatology* 34, no. 3 (2007): 548–55.

Hsu, C.C. et al. "Use of Nonsteroidal Anti-Inflammatory Drugs and Risk of Chronic Kidney Disease in Subjects with Hypertension: Nationwide Longitudinal Cohort Study." *Hypertension.* Published electronically July 13, 2015.

Jaeschke, H. "Acetaminophen: Dose-Dependent Drug Hepatotoxicity and Acute Liver Failure in Patients." *Digestive Diseases* 33, no. 4 (2015): 464–71.

Lip, G.Y. "Nonsteroidal Anti-Inflammatory Drugs and Bleeding Risk in Anticoagulated Patients with Atrial Fibrillation." *Expert*

Review of Cardiovascular Therapy 13, no. 9 (Jul. 21, 2015): 1–3.

Martini, D.I. et al. "Serotonin Syndrome Following Metaxalone Overdose and Therapeutic Use of a Selective Serotonin Reuptake Inhibitor." *Clinical Toxicology* 53, no. 3 (Mar. 2015): 185–7.

Pearlman, B.L., and R. Gambhir. "Salicylate Intoxication: A Clinical Review." *Postgraduate Medicine* 121, no. 4 (Jul. 2009): 162–8.

Tarraga Lopez, P.J. et al. "Primary and Secondary Prevention of Colorectal Cancer." *Clinical Medical Insights: Gastroenterology* 7 (Jul. 14, 2014): 33–46.

Warner, M. et al. "Drug Poisoning Deaths in the United States, 1980–2008." *NCHS Data Brief No. 81* (Dec. 2011).

Checklist 9

Bohm, N.M. et al. "Hemarthrosis in a Patient on Warfarin Receiving Ceftaroline: A Case Report and Brief Review of Cephalosporin Interactions with Warfarin." *The Annals of Pharmacotherapy* 46, nos. 7–8 (Jul.–Aug. 2012): e19.

Bushra, R. et al. "Food-Drug Interactions." *Oman Medical Journal* 26, no. 2 (Mar. 2011): 77–83.

Cohen, J.S. "Peripheral Neuropathy Associated with Fluoroquinolones." *The Annals of Pharmacotherapy* 35, no. 12 (Dec. 2001): 1540–7.

Cots, J.M. et al. "Recommendations for Management of Acute Pharyngitis in Adults." *Atencion primaria* 66, no. 3 (May 26, 2015): 159–70.

Dickinson, B.D. et al. "Drug Interactions Between Oral Contraceptives and Antibiotics." *Obstetrics and Gynecology* 98, no. 5 (Nov. 2001): 853–60.

Gandhi, S. et al. "Calcium-Channel Blocker-Clarithromycin Drug Interactions and Acute Kidney Injury." *JAMA* 310, no. 23 (Dec. 18, 2013): 2544–53.

Jayasagar, G. et al. "Effect of Cephalexin on the Pharmacokinetics of Metformin in Healthy Human Volunteers." *Drug Metabolism and Drug Interactions* 19, no. 1 (2002): 41–8.

Ming, E.E. et al. "Concomitant Use of Statins and CYP3A4 Inhibitors in Administrative

Claims and Electronic Medical Records Databases." *Journal of Clinical Lipidology* 2, no. 6 (Dec. 2008): 453–63.

Singh, A. et al. "Reversible Interstitial Lung Disease with Prolonged Use of Nitrofurantoin: Do the Benefits Outweigh the Risks?" *Lung India* 30, no. 3 (Jul. 2013): 212–4.

van der Linden, P.D. et al. "Increased Risk of Achilles Tendon Rupture with Quinolone Antibacterial Use, Especially in Elderly Patients Taking Oral Corticosteroids." *Archives of Internal Medicine* 163, no. 15 (2003): 1801–7.

Zarychanski, R. et al. "Pharmacokinetic Interaction Between Methotrexate and Piperacillin/Tazobactam Resulting in Prolonged Toxic Concentrations of Methotrexate." *Journal of Antimicrobial Chemotherapy* 58(1) (2006): 228–30.

Checklist 10

Anderson, J.W. et al. "Health Benefits of Dietary Fiber." *Nutrition Reviews* 67, no. 4 (Apr. 2009): 188–205.

Bain, L.K. et al. "The Relationship Between Dietary Magnesium Intake, Stroke and Its Major Risk Factors, Blood Pressure and Cholesterol, in the EPIC-Norfolk Cohort." *International Journal of Cardiology* 196 (Oct. 1, 2015): 108–14.

Bolten, W.W. et al. "The Safety and Efficacy of an Enzyme Combination in Managing Knee Osteoarthritis Pain in Adults: A Randomized, Double-Blind, Placebo-Controlled Trial." *Arthritis* 2015 (2015): Article ID 251521.

Conrozier, T. et al. "A Complex of Three Natural Anti-Inflammatory Agents Provides Relief of Osteoarthritis Pain." *Alternative Therapies in Health and Medicine* 20, suppl. 1 (Winter 2014): 32–7.

Cordero, M.D. et al. "Can Coenzyme Q_{10} Improve Clinical and Molecular Parameters in Fibromyalgia?" *Antioxidants and Redox Signaling* 9, no. 12 (Oct. 2013): 1356–61.

Fabian, A. et al. "The Effect of Daily Consumption of Probiotic and Conventional Yoghurt on Oxidant and Antioxidant Parameters in
Plasma of Young Healthy Women." *International Journal for Vitamin and Nutrition Research* 77 (2007): 79–88.

Flanigan, R. et al. "D-Ribose Aids Fatigue in Aging Adults." *Journal of Alternative and Complementary Medicine* 16, no. 5 (May 2010): 529–30.

Henriksen, E.J. "Exercise Training and the Antioxidant Alpha-Lipoic Acid in the Treatment of Insulin Resistance and Type 2 Diabetes." *Free Radical Biology and Medicine* 40, no. 1 (Jan. 1, 2006): 3–12.

Hilmi, B.A. et al. "Use of Newly Available Febuxostat in a Case of Chronic Tophaceous Gout Contraindicated to Allopurinol and Probenecid." *Medical Journal of Malaysia* 67, no. 1 (Feb. 2012): 125–6.

Ho, M.J., A. Bellusci, and J.M. Wright. "Blood Pressure Lowering Efficacy of Coenzyme Q_{10} for Primary Hypertension." *Cochrane Database of Systematic Reviews* (Oct. 7, 2009).

Howatson, G. et al. "Influence of Tart Cherry Juice on Indices of Recovery Following Marathon Running." *Scandinavian Journal of Medicine and Science in Sports* 20, no. 6 (Dec. 2010): 843–52.

Kimmatkar, N. et al. "Efficacy and Tolerability of Boswellia Serrata Extract in Treatment of Osteoarthritis of Knee–A Randomized Double Blind Placebo Controlled Trial." *Phytomedicine* 10, no. 1 (Jan. 2003): 3–7.

Knuesel, O. et al. "Arnica Montana Gel in Osteoarthritis of the Knee: An Open, Multicenter Clinical Trial." *Advances in Therapy* 19, no. 5 (Sep.–Oct. 2002): 209–18.

Kuehl, K.S. "Cherry Juice Targets Antioxidant Potential and Pain Relief." *Medicine & Sports Science* 59 (2012): 86–93.

Kuehl, K.S. et al. "Efficacy of Tart Cherry Juice in Reducing Muscle Pain During Running: A Randomized Controlled Trial." *Journal of the International Society of Sports Nutrition* 7 (May 7, 2010): 17.

Kuptniratsaikul, V. et al. "Efficacy and Safety of Curcuma Domestica Extracts Compared with Ibuprofen in Patients with Knee Osteoarthritis: A Multicenter Study." *Clinical Interventions in Aging* 9 (Mar. 20, 2014): 451–8.

Lomax, A.R. et al. "Probiotics, Immune Function, Infection and Inflammation: A Review of the Evidence from Studies Conducted in Humans." *Current Pharmaceutical Design* 15, no. 13 (2009): 1428–518.

Maes, M. et al. "Lower Plasma Coenzyme Q_{10} in Depression: A Marker for Treatment Resistance and Chronic Fatigue in Depression and a Risk Factor to Cardiovascular Disorder in That Illness." *Neuroendocrinology Letters* 30, no. 4 (2009): 462–9.

Malina, D.M. et al. "Additive Effects of Plant Sterols Supplementation in Addition to Different Lipid-Lowering Regimens." *Journal of Clinical Lipidology* 9, no. 4 (Jul.–Aug. 2015): 542–52.

Panossian, A. et al. "Evidence-Based Efficacy of Adaptogens in Fatigue, and Molecular Mechanisms Related to Their Stress-Protective Activity." *Current Clinical Pharmacology* 4, no. 3 (Sep. 2009): 198–219.

Papanas, N. et al. "Efficacy of Alpha Lipoic Acid in Diabetic Neuropathy." *Expert Opinion on Pharmacotherapy* 15, no. 18 (Dec. 2014): 2721–31.

Regal, R.E. et al. "Urinary Tract Infections in Extended Care Facilities: Preventive Management Strategies." *The Consultant Pharmacist* 21, no. 5 (May 2006): 400–9.

Ried, K. et al. "Aged Garlic Extract Reduces Blood Pressure in Hypertensives: A Dose-Response Trial." *European Journal of Clinical Nutrition* 67, no. 1 (Jan. 2013): 64–70.

Rondanelli, M. et al. "The Effect of Melatonin, Magnesium, and Zinc on Primary Insomnia in Long-Term Care Facility Residents in Italy: A Double-Blind, Placebo-Controlled Clinical Trial." *Journal of the American Geriatrics Society* 59, no. 1 (Jan. 2011): 82–90.

Ross, S.M. "Osteoarthritis: A Proprietary Arnica Gel Is Found to Be as Effective as Ibuprofen Gel in Osteoarthritis of the Hands." *Holistic Nursing Practice* 22, no. 4 (Jul.–Aug. 2008): 237–9.

Rostami, A. et al. "High-Cocoa Polyphenol-Rich Chocolate Improves Blood Pressure in Patients with Diabetes and Hypertension." *ARYA Atherosclerosis* 11, no. 1 (Jan. 2015): 21–9.

Russell, I.J. et al. "Treatment of Fibromyalgia Syndrome with Super Malic: A Randomized, Double Blind, Placebo Controlled, Crossover Pilot Study." *Journal of Rheumatology* 22, no. 5 (May 1995): 953–8.

Sahebkar, A. "Why Is It Necessary to Translate Curcumin into Clinical Practice for the Prevention and Treatment of Metabolic Syndrome?" *Biofactors* 39, no. 2 (Mar.–Apr. 2013): 197–208.

Simopoulos, A.P. "Omega-3 Fatty Acids in Inflammation and Autoimmune Diseases." *Journal of the American College of Nutrition* 21, no. 6 (Dec. 2002): 495–505.

Susalit, E. et al. "Olive (*Olea europaea*) Leaf Extract Effective in Patients with Stage-1 Hypertension: Comparison with Captopril." *Phytomedicine* 18, no. 4 (Feb. 15, 2011): 251–8.

Tsuneki, H. et al. "Protective Effects of Coenzyme Q_{10} Against Angiotensin II-Induced Oxidative Stress in Human Umbilical Vein Endothelial Cells." *European Journal of Pharmacology* 701, nos. 1–3 (Feb. 15, 2013): 218–27.

Vicariotto, F. "Effectiveness of an Association of a Cranberry Dry Extract, D-Mannose, and the Two Microorganisms *Lactobacillus plantarum* LP01 and *Lactobacillus paracasei* LPC09 in Women Affected by Cystitis: A Pilot Study." *Journal of Clinical Gastroenterology* 48, suppl. 1 (Nov.–Dec. 2014): S96–101.

Woods, C.A. et al. "Febuxostat (Uloric), A New Treatment Option for Gout." *Pharmacy and Therapeutics* 35, no. 2 (Feb. 2010): 82–85.

Zhang, Y. et al. "Cherry Consumption and Decreased Risk of Recurrent Gout Attacks." *Arthritis and Rheumatism* 64, no. 12 (Dec. 2012): 4004–11.

Ziegler, D. et al. "Treatment of Symptomatic Diabetic Polyneuropathy with the Antioxidant Alpha-Lipoic Acid: A Meta-Analysis." *Diabetic Medicine* 21, no. 2 (Feb. 2004): 114–21.

Zuhl, M. et al. "The Effects of Acute Oral Glutamine Supplementation on Exercise-Induced Gastrointestinal Permeability and Heat Shock Protein Expression in Peripheral Blood Mononuclear Cells." *Cell Stress and Chaperones* 20, no. 1 (Jan. 2015): 85–93.

Index

About the Authors

Dr. Richard W. Snyder is a nephrologist on the staff of St. Luke's University Hospital Network and Easton Hospital in Pennsylvania. He received his medical degree from Philadelphia College of Osteopathic Medicine and has been in practice for more than eleven years. Dr. Snyder is also the author of *Medical Dosage Calculations for Dummies* (Wiley), *Adrenal Fatigue for Dummies* (Wiley), *Physician Assistant National Certifying Exam for Dummies* (Wiley), as well as *What You Must Know About Kidney Disease* (Square One), *What You Must Know About Dialysis* (Square One), and the recently released *What You Must Know About Liver Disease* (Square One). He is the associate program director of the Internal Medicine Residency Program at Easton Hospital. Dr. Snyder lives in Easton, Pennsylvania.

Dr. Koroush Khalighi, a pioneering integrative cardiologist and electrophysiologist, is the director at the Cardiac Electrophysiology Lab, as well as the Director of Clinical Research, at Easton Hospital in Pennsylvania. He has utilized a personalized medication approach for the treatment of hundreds of patients and is the principal clinical investigator for more than thirty clinical studies, several of which have been sponsored by the National Institute of Health. He was the recipient of the American Heart Association's Cardiovascular Research Award in 2000. Dr. Khalighi lives in Easton, Pennsylvania.